A Parcel of Purple

By Emma Rose Sparrow

Publish Date: February 13, 2015

Editor-in-Chief: Connor Chagnon
Sterling Elle Publishing
Bradford, Massachusetts
ISBN-10: 1517419506
ISBN-13: 978-1517419509

A PARCEL OF PURPLE

An Emma Rose Sparrow Book

A PARCEL OF PURPLE is a collection of amazing photos - with accompanying text - that have one thing in common: the color purple!

You may be surprised how much purple exists in the world. From lush purple fields of lavender to the shimmering wings of the Purple Emperor butterfly, this book brings the color purple to life.

If you are an adult bookworm who enjoys exquisite photos, this book is for you!

It is hoped that you find this book worthy of adding to your collection.

Enjoy your read!

OTHER BOOKS IN THIS SERIES BY EMMA ROSE SPARROW

A Bevy of Blue

A Year's Worth of Yellow

A Gathering of Green

A Potpourri of Pink

A Reservoir of Red

A World of White

An Ocean of Orange

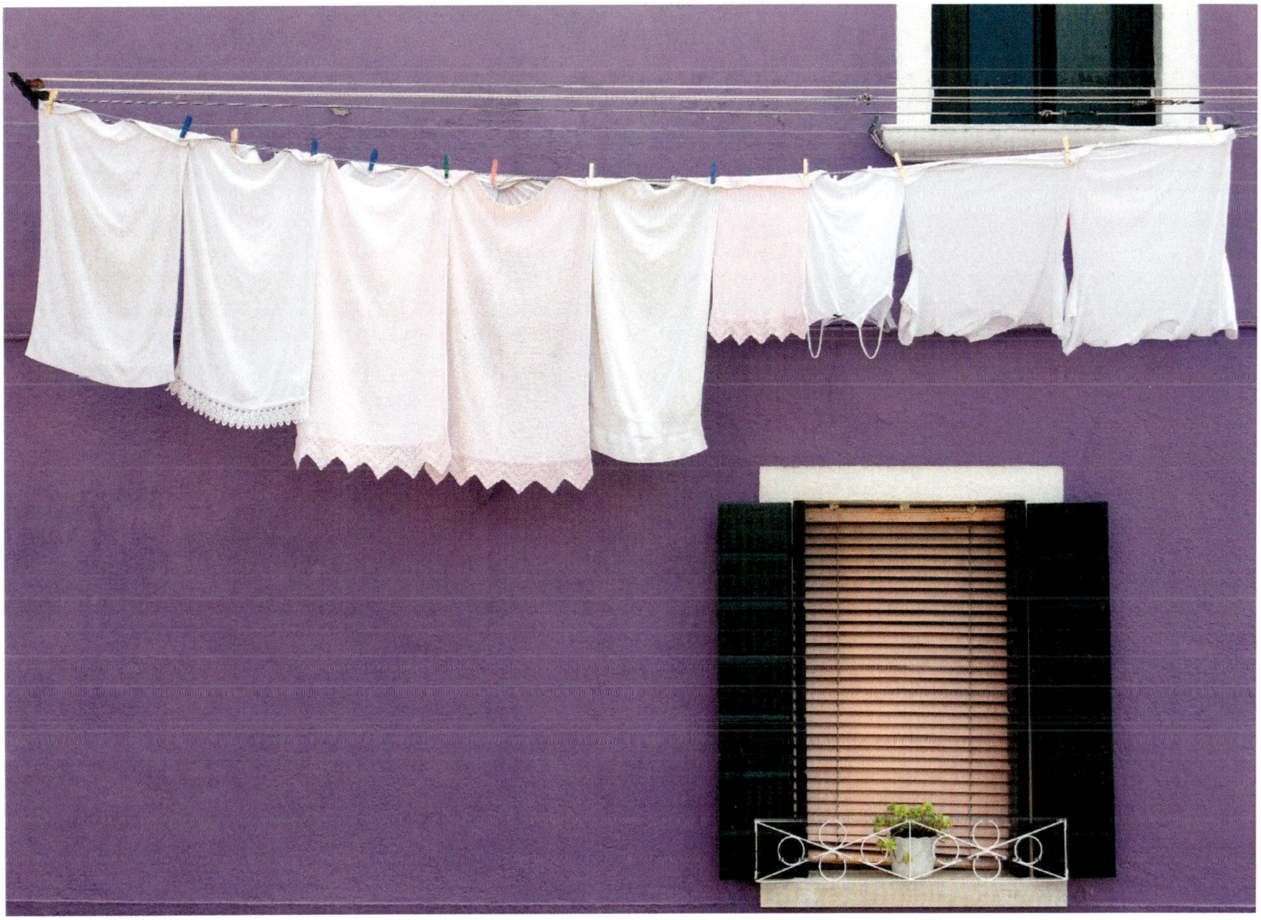

A clothesline is strung in front of a purple house in Burano, an Italian island.

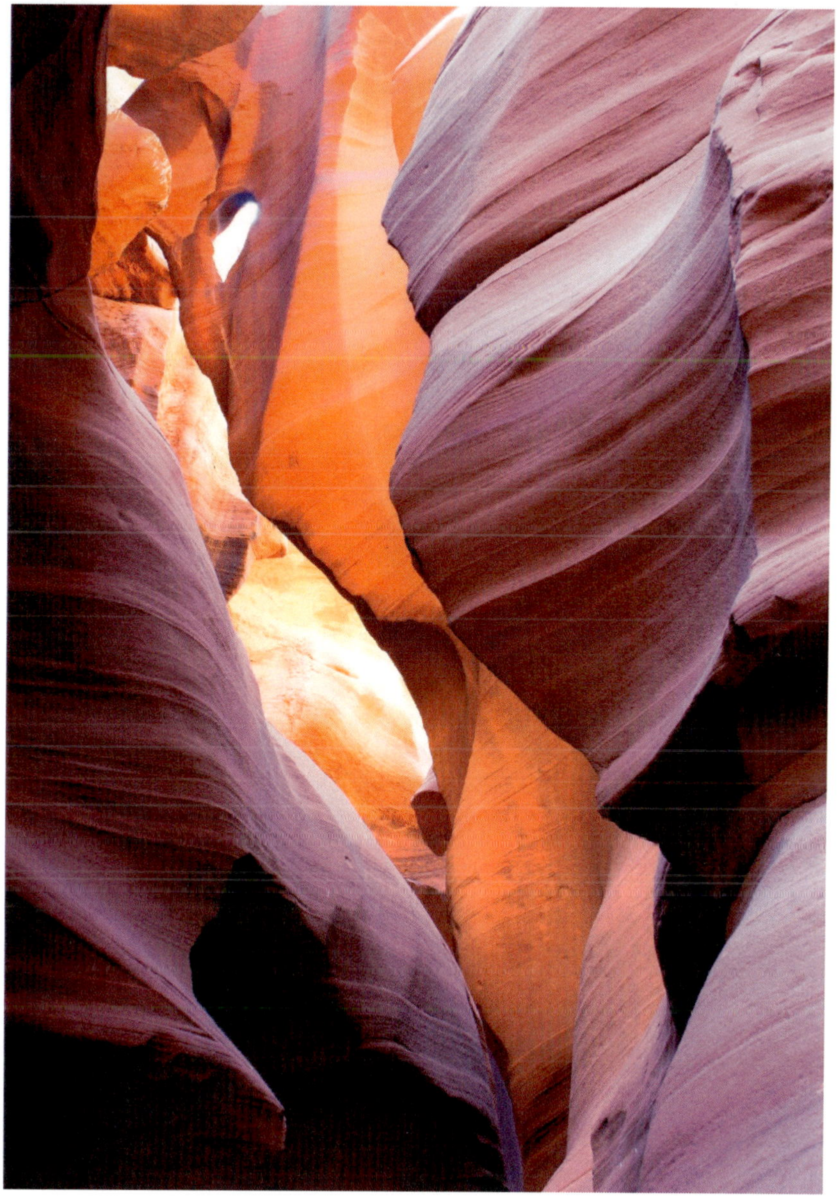

Shaded areas of these rock formations in Antelope Canyon, Arizona, appear as a muted purple.

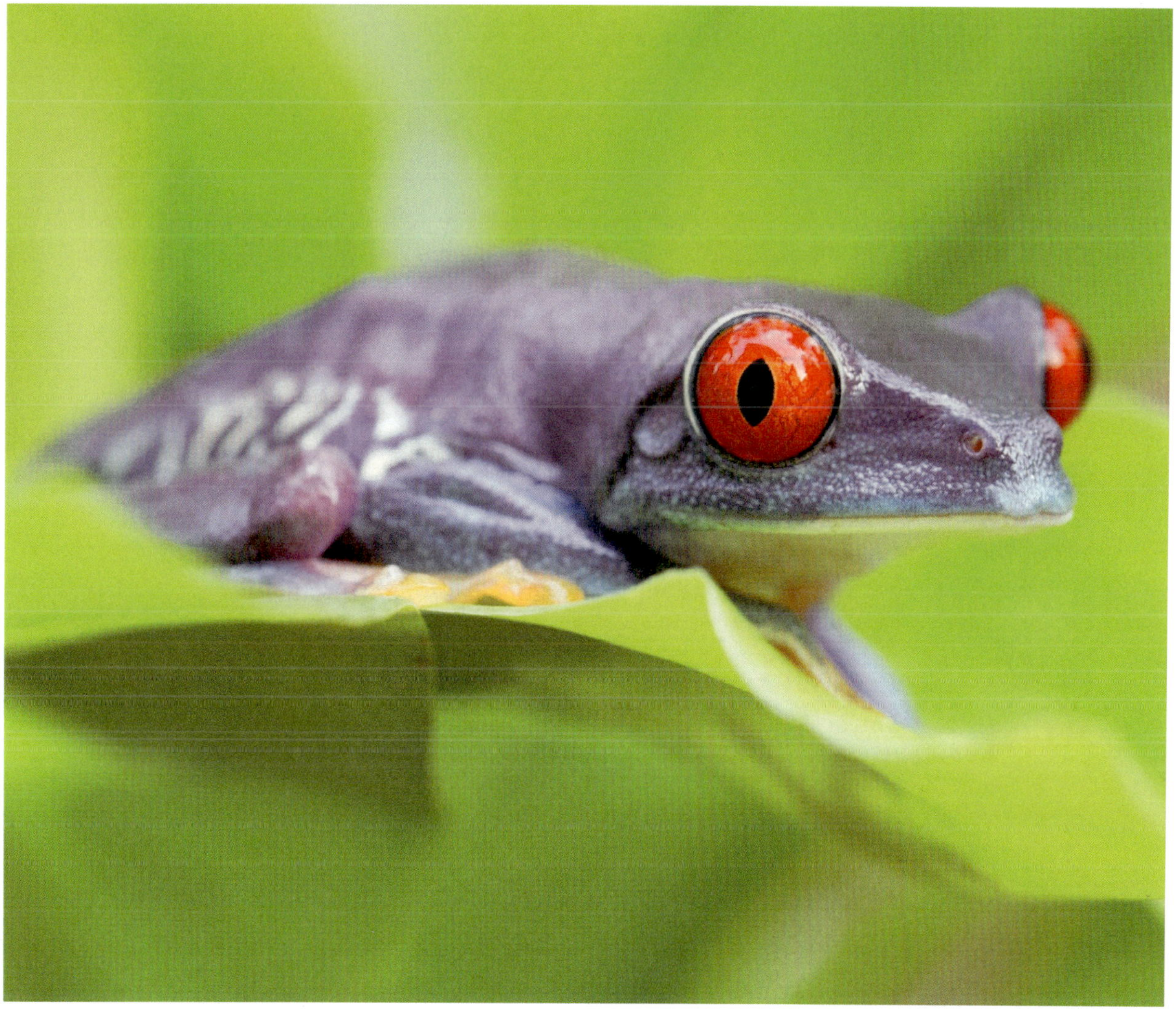

A purple Red Eyed tree frog in Costa Rica.

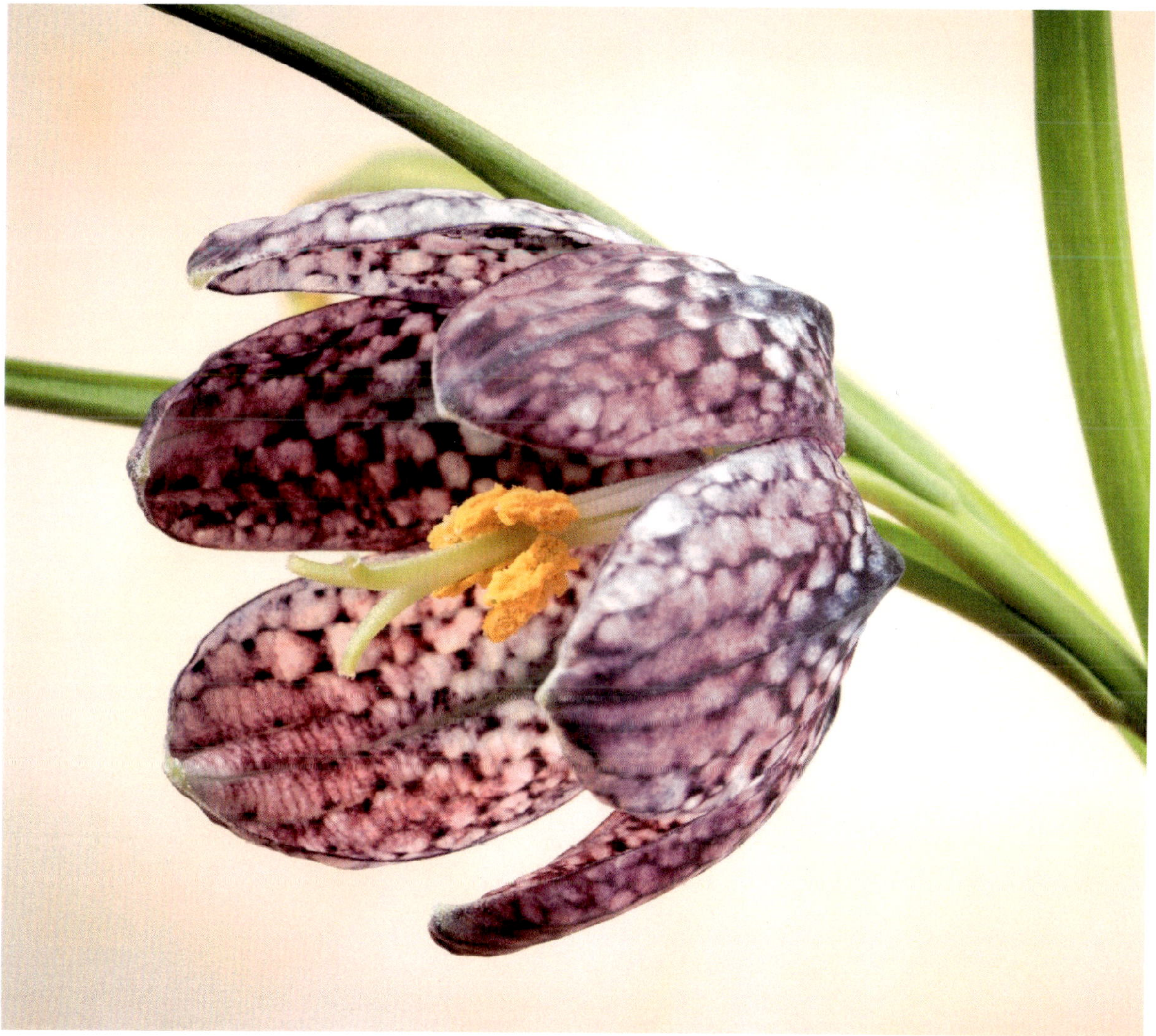

This purple chess flower is an endangered species in many areas.

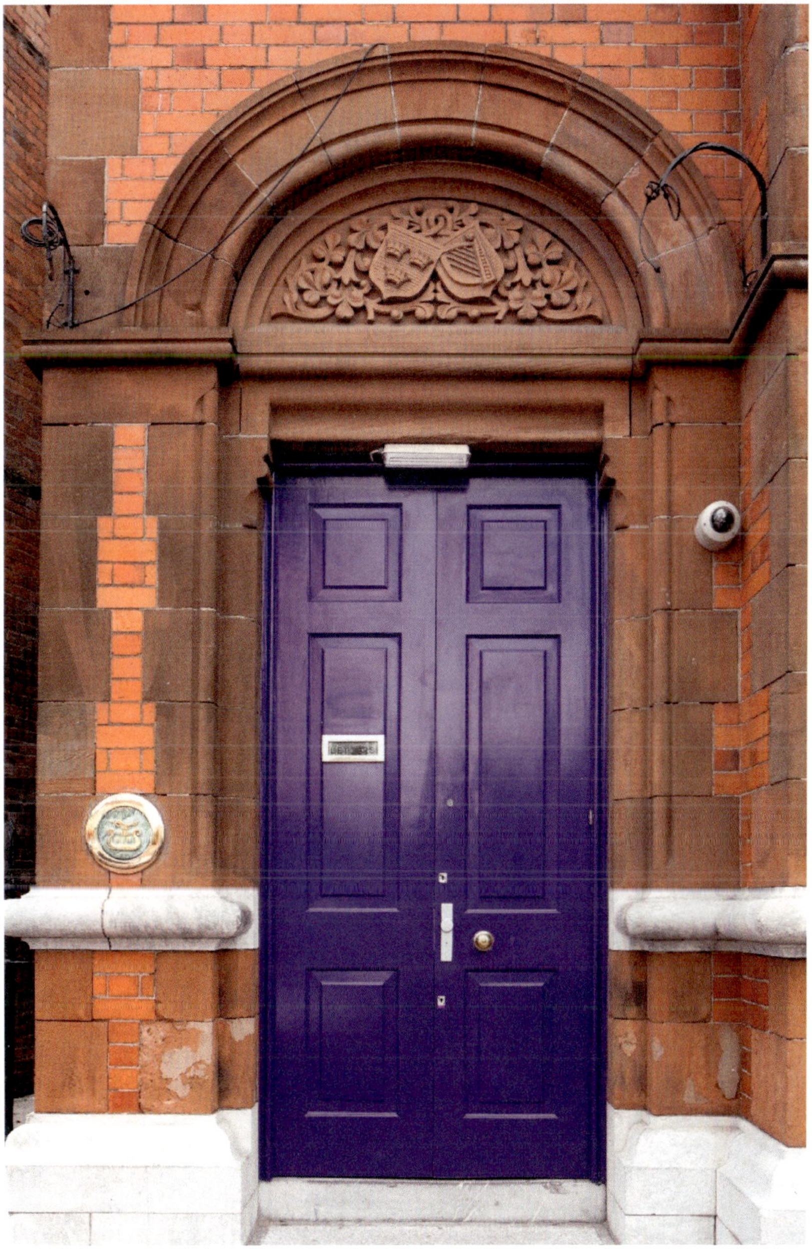

This purple door marks the entrance to a bank in Ireland.

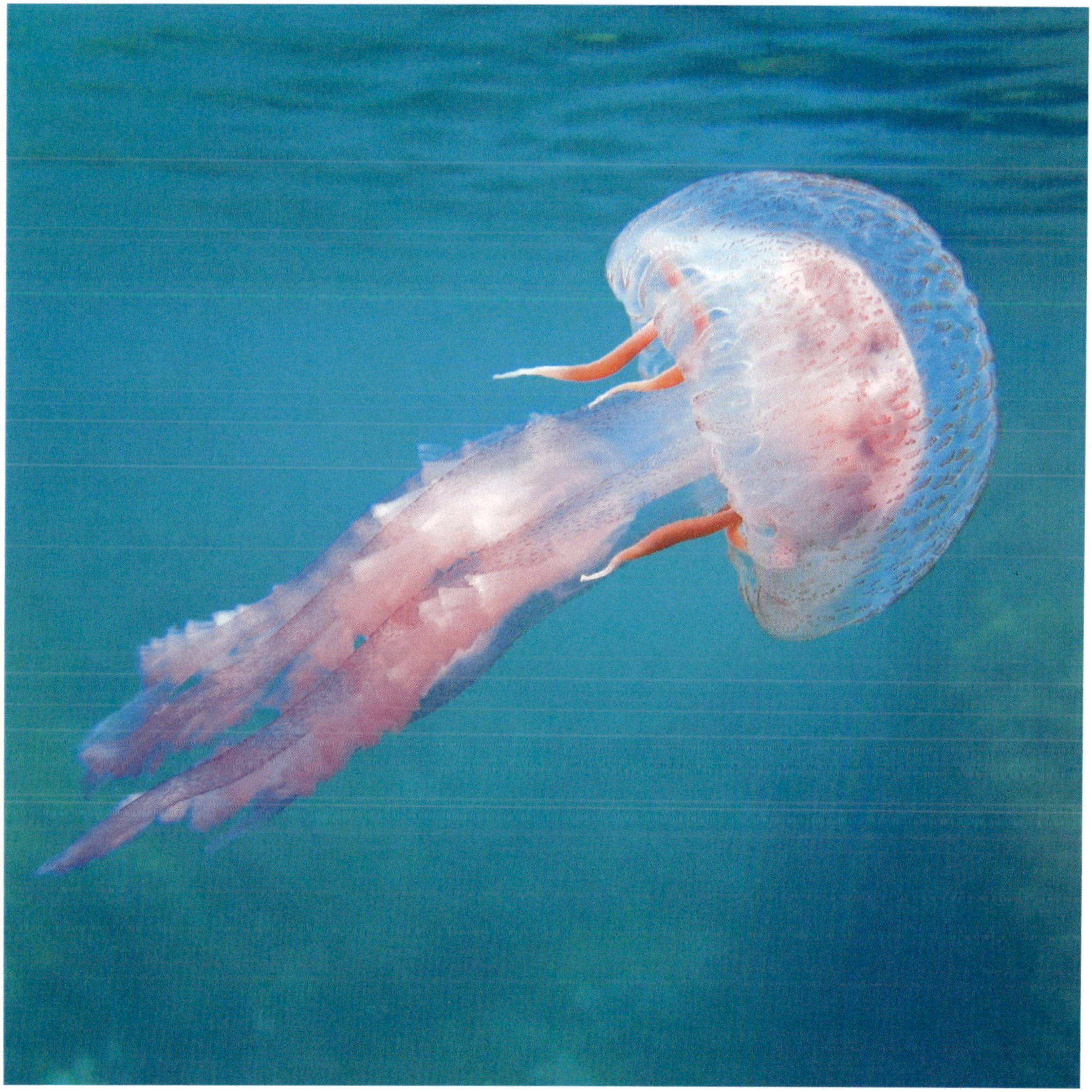

This purple jellyfish has many names, including the Mauve Stinger.
Here, a photo is snapped off the coast of Hawaii.

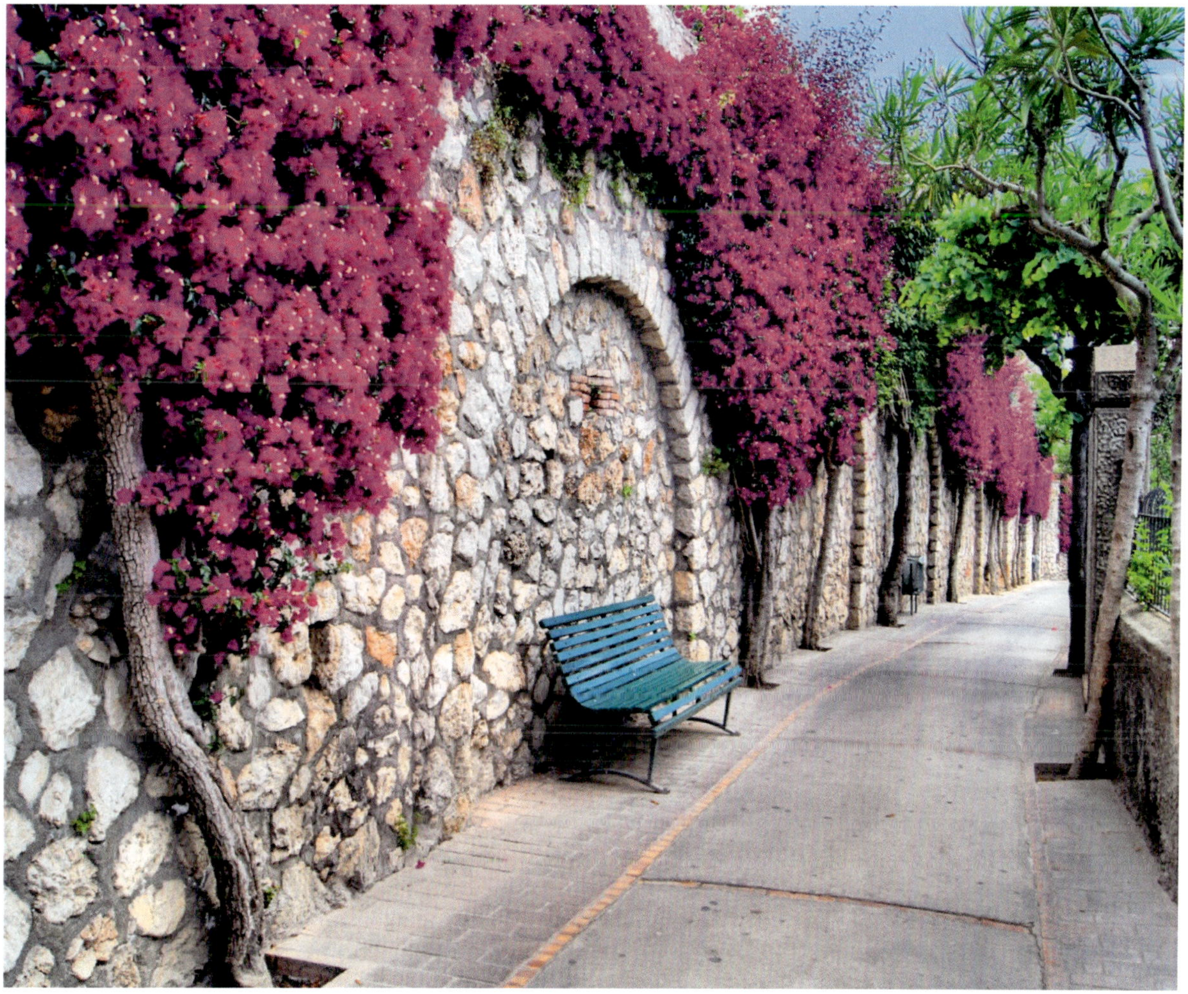

Vibrant purple flowers drape over the walls of a pathway in Capri, Italy.

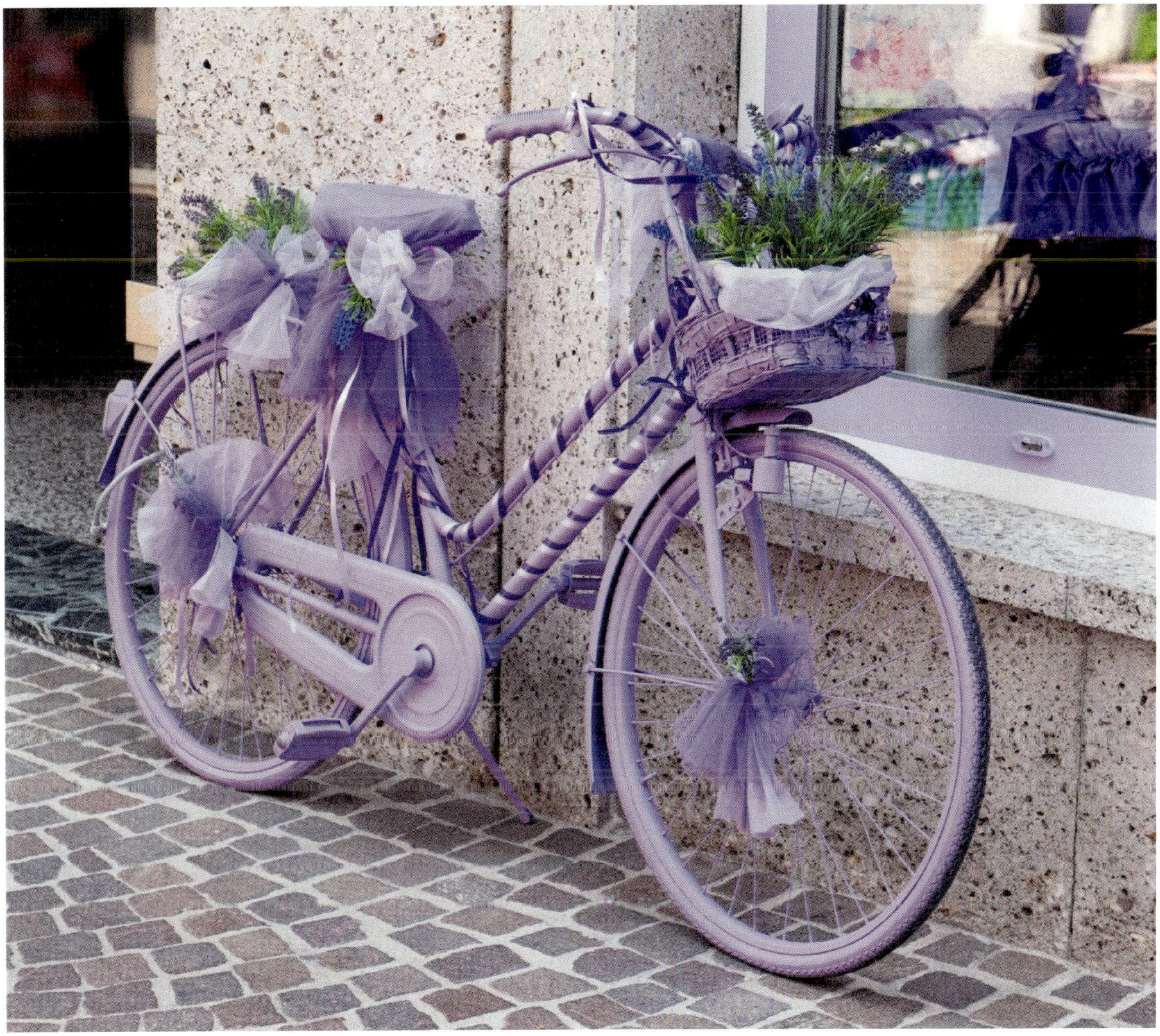

A decorated purple bicycle outside of a café in England.

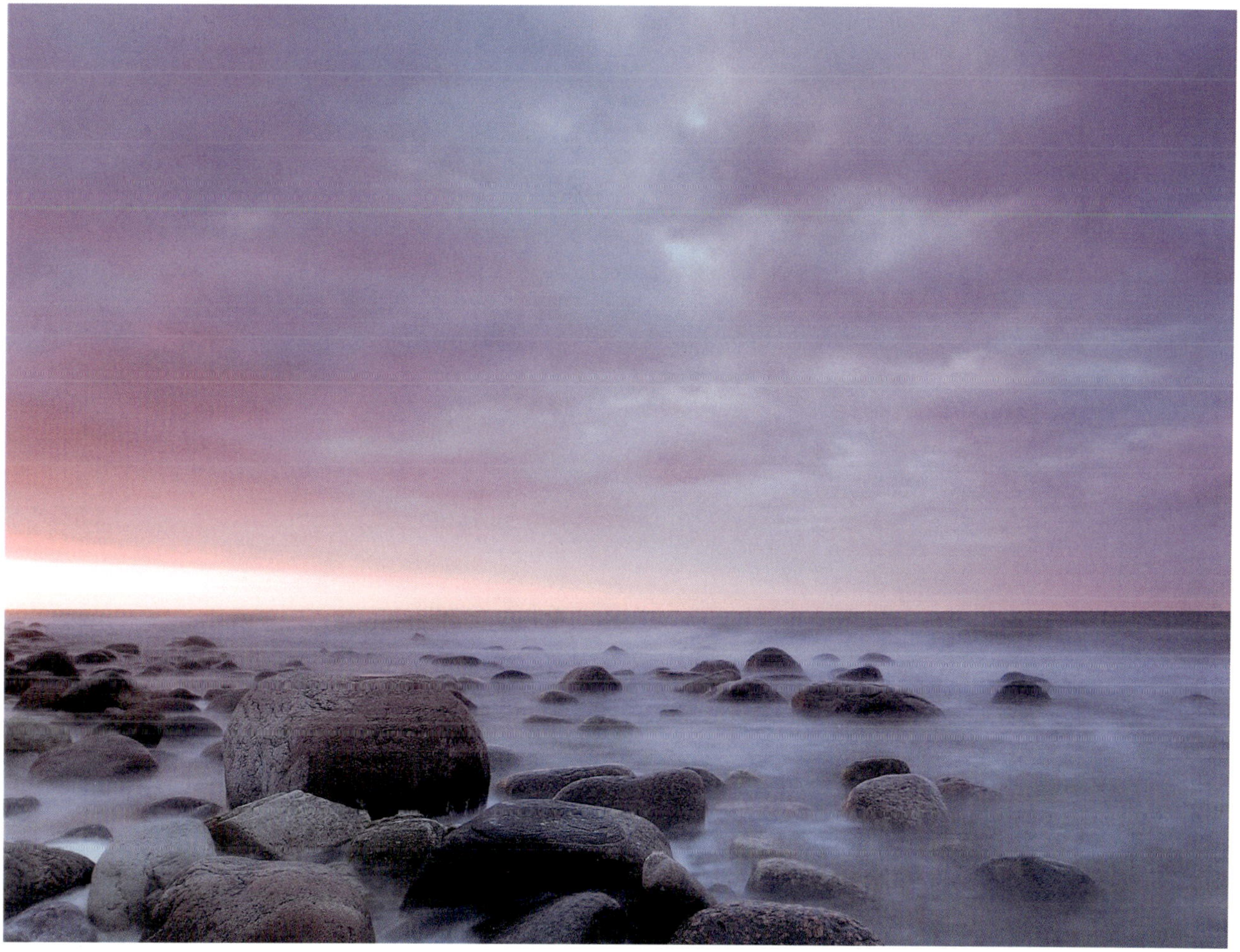

From the sky to the fog-covered rocks, purple reigns in this sunrise over the Swedish coastline.

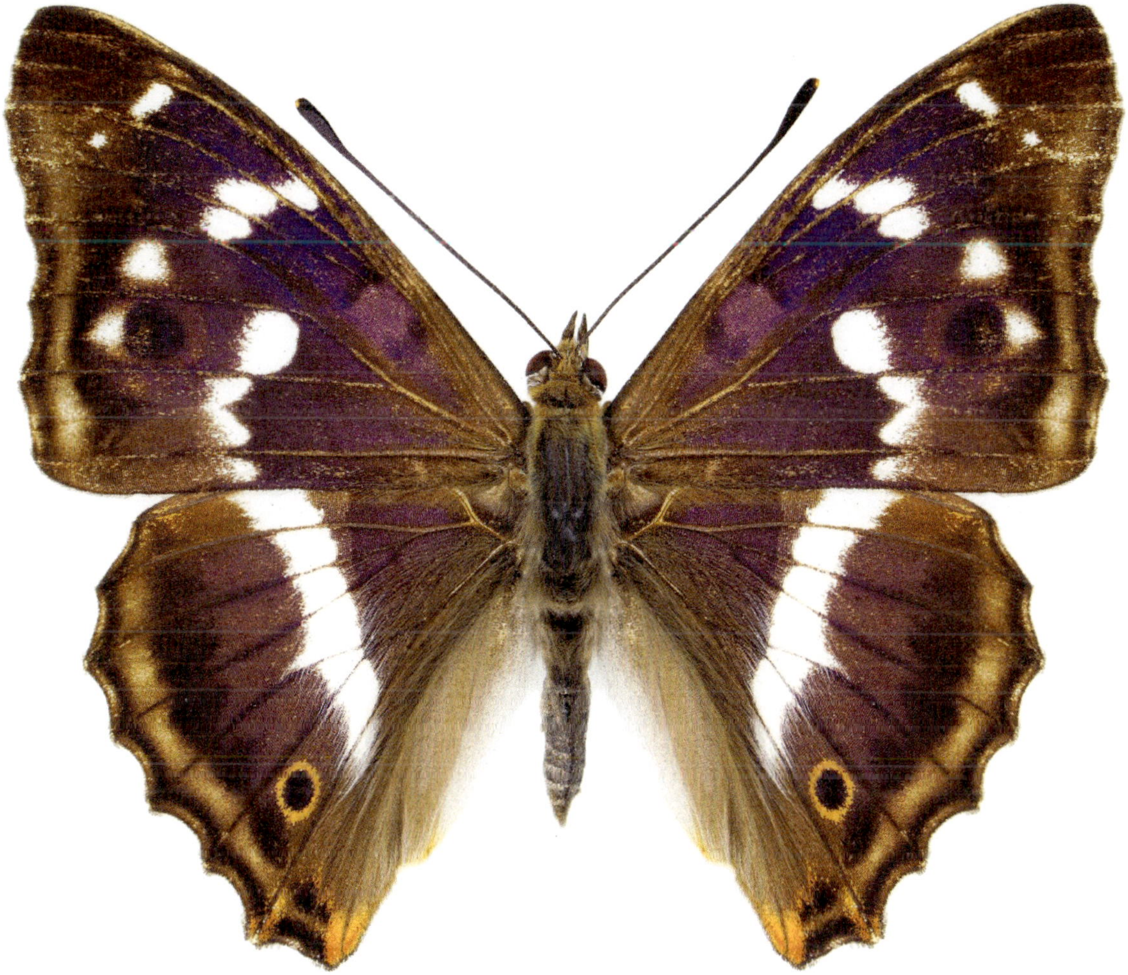

This is the Purple Emperor butterfly.
Only the males have these shimmering purple markings.

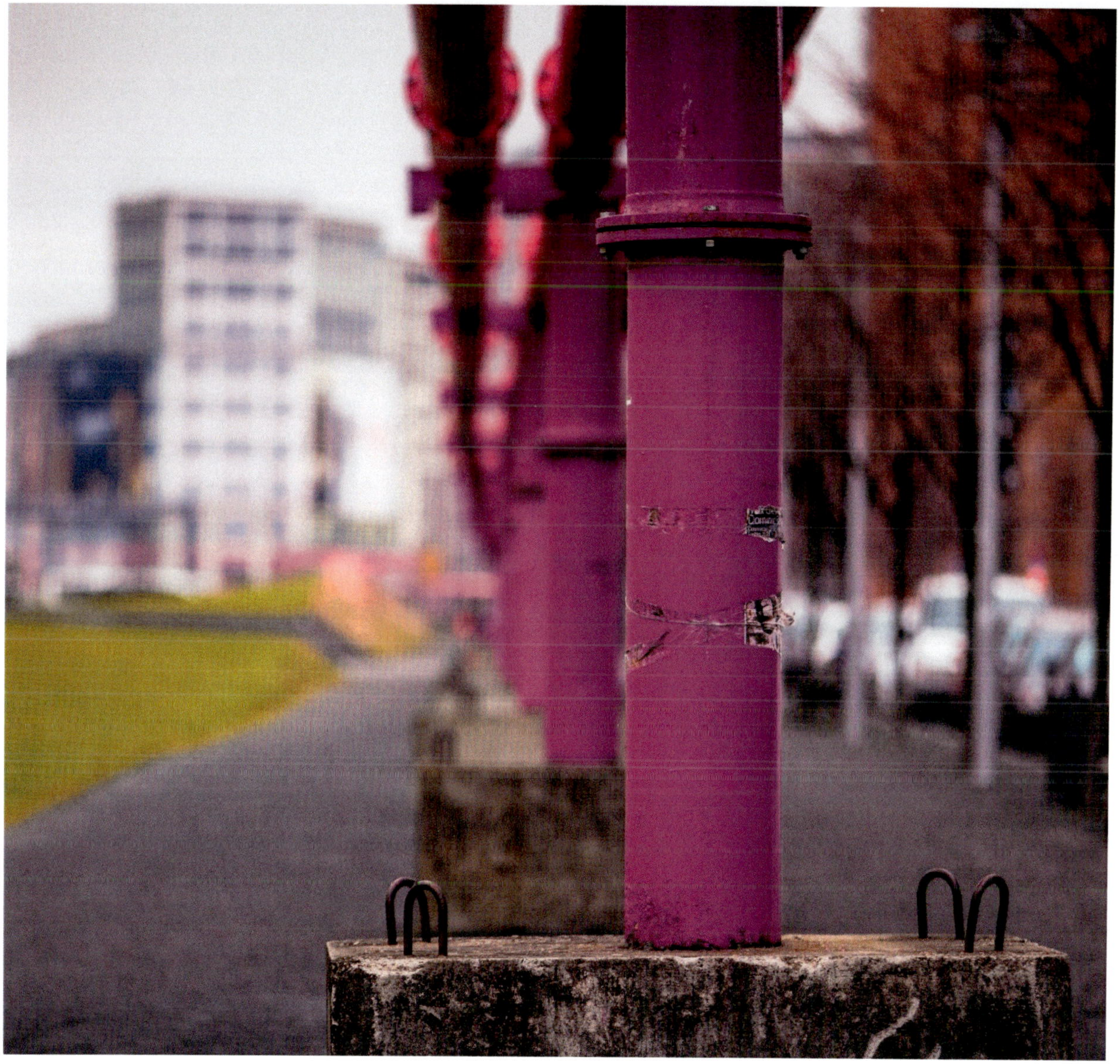

These utility poles in Belgium were painted a lively purple.

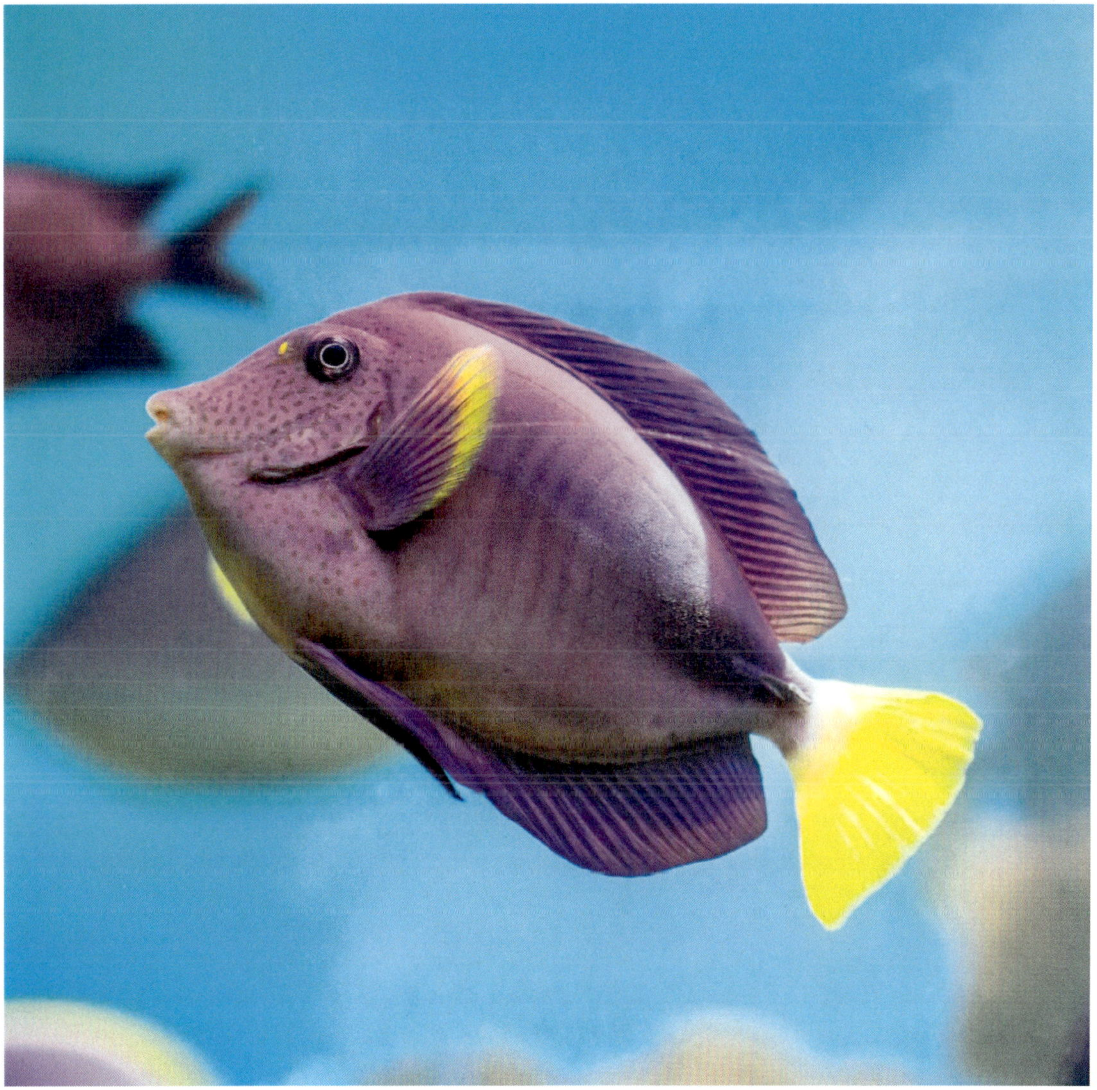

The Yellowfin Surgeonfish tends to develop a deeper purple as it ages.

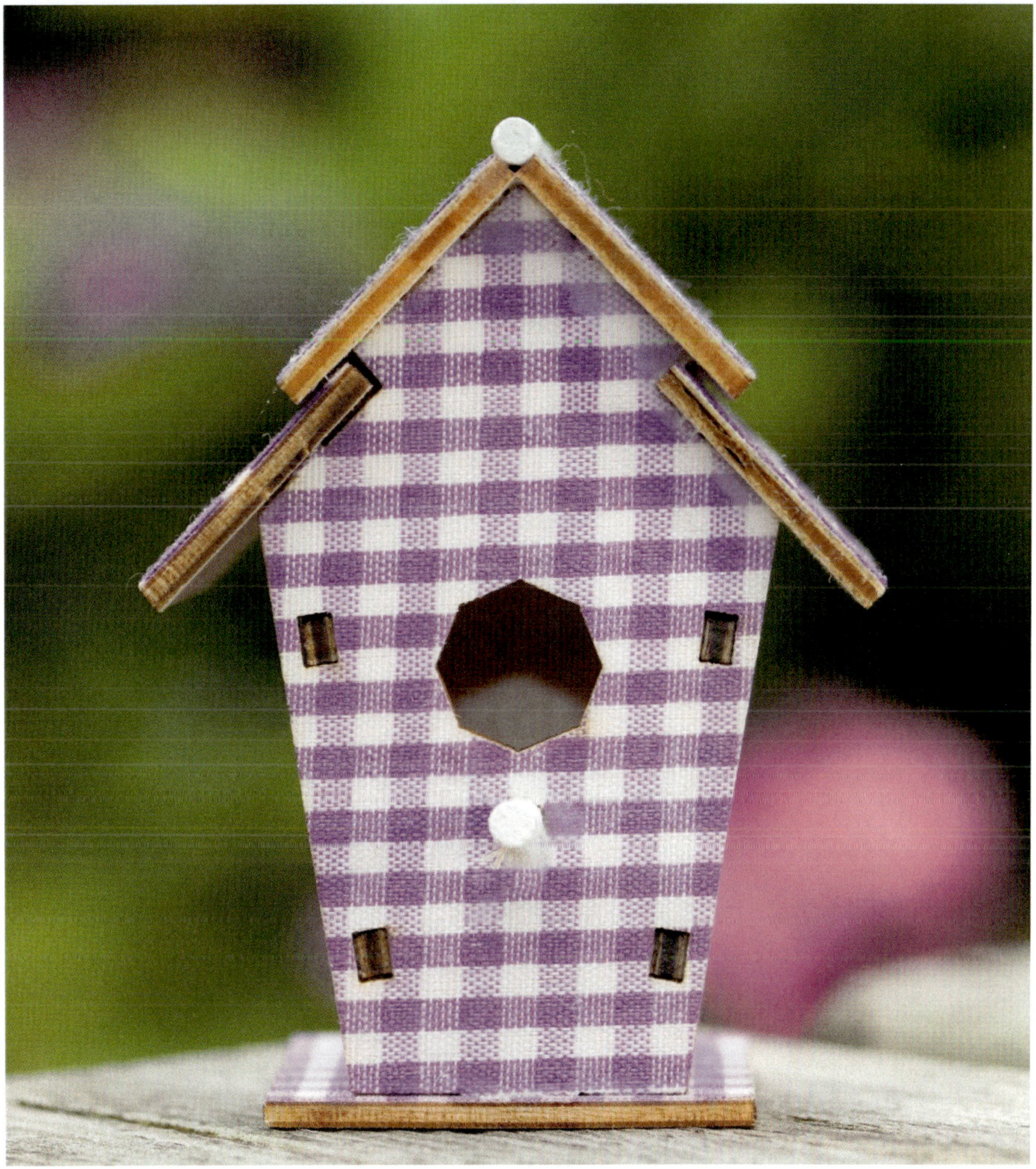

A homemade bird house covered with white and purple fabric.

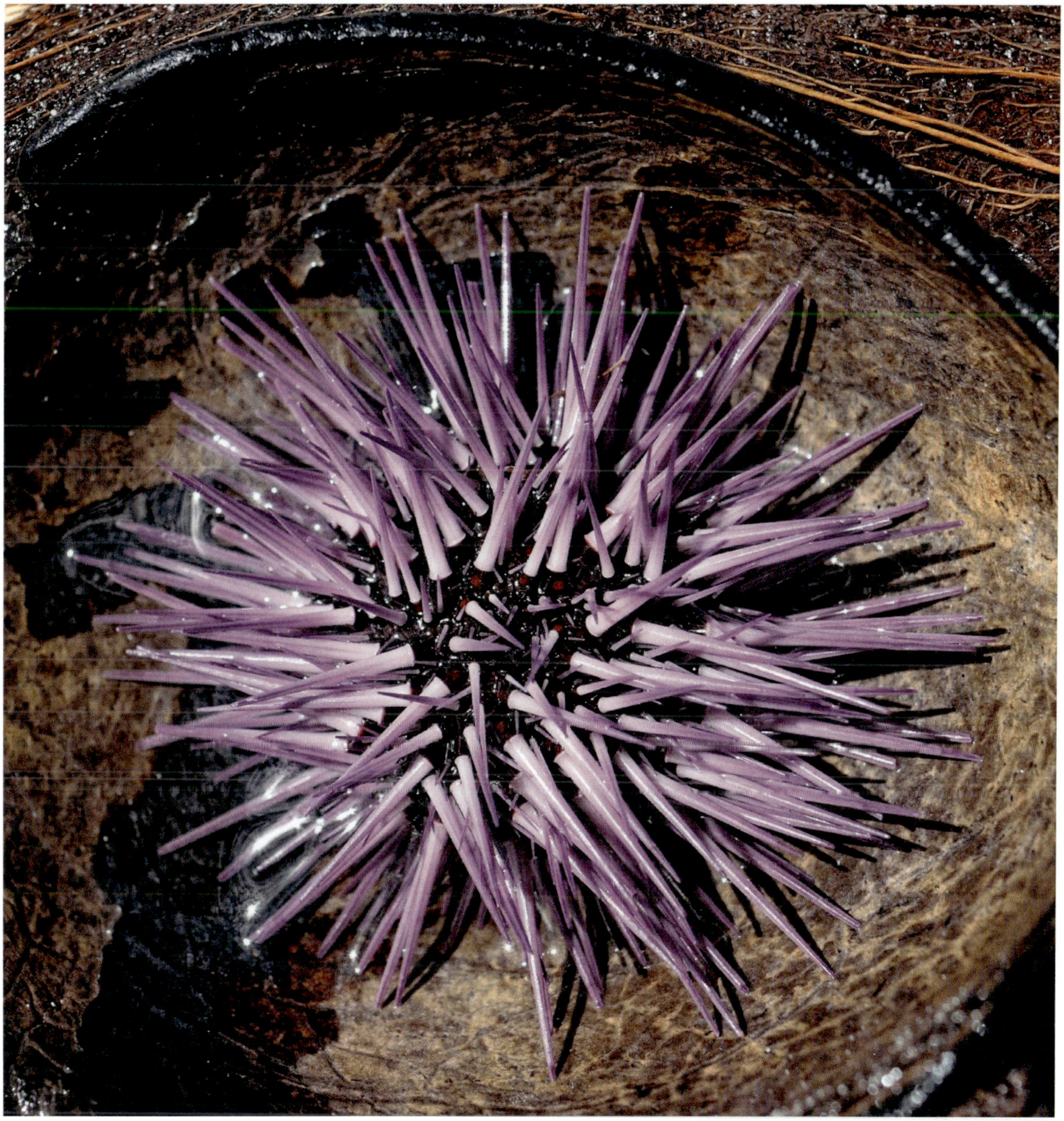

A purple sea urchin in coconut shell.

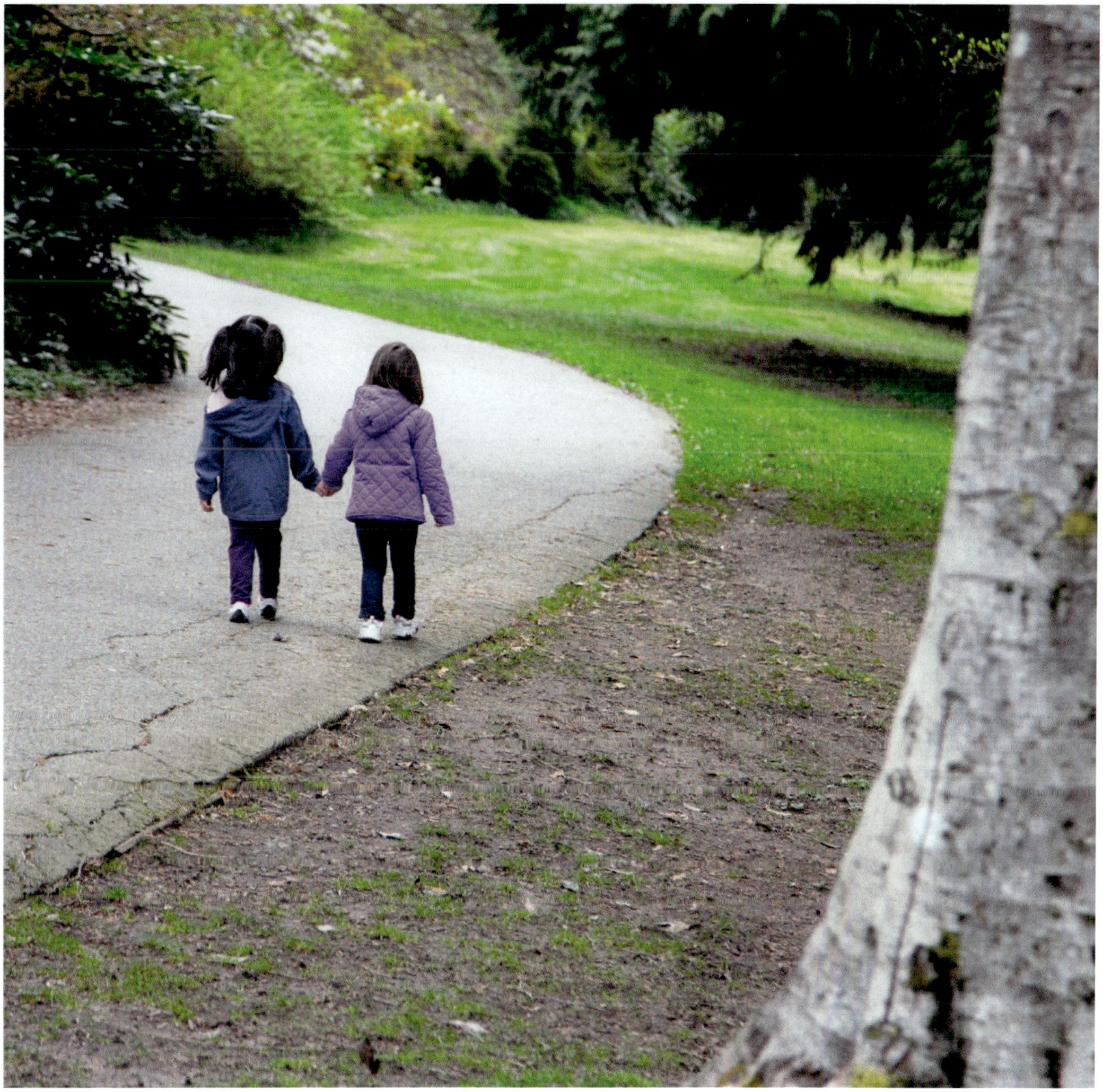

In Scotland, young sisters dressed in purple hold hands.

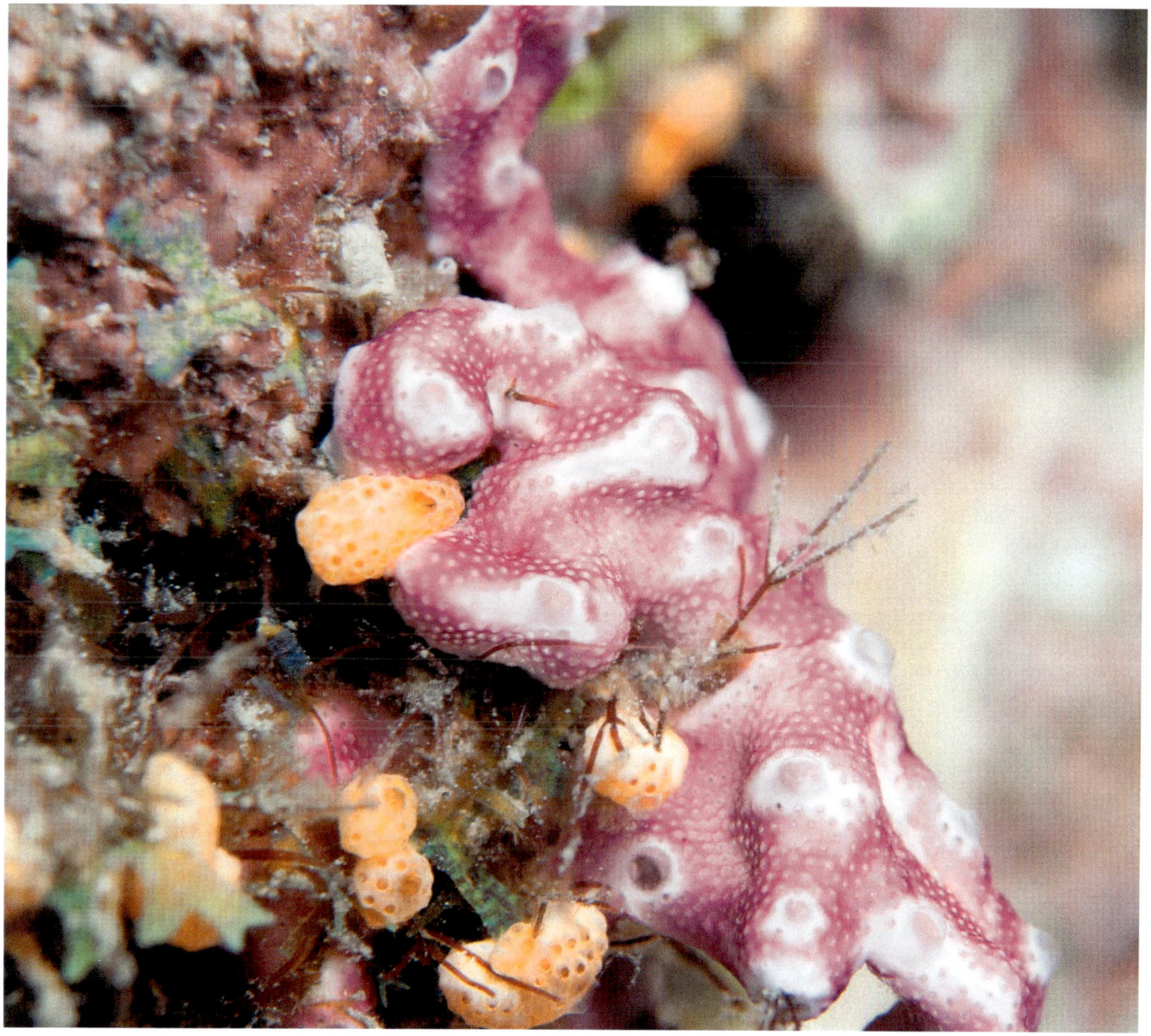

Delicate purple and white coral off the coast of St. John island.

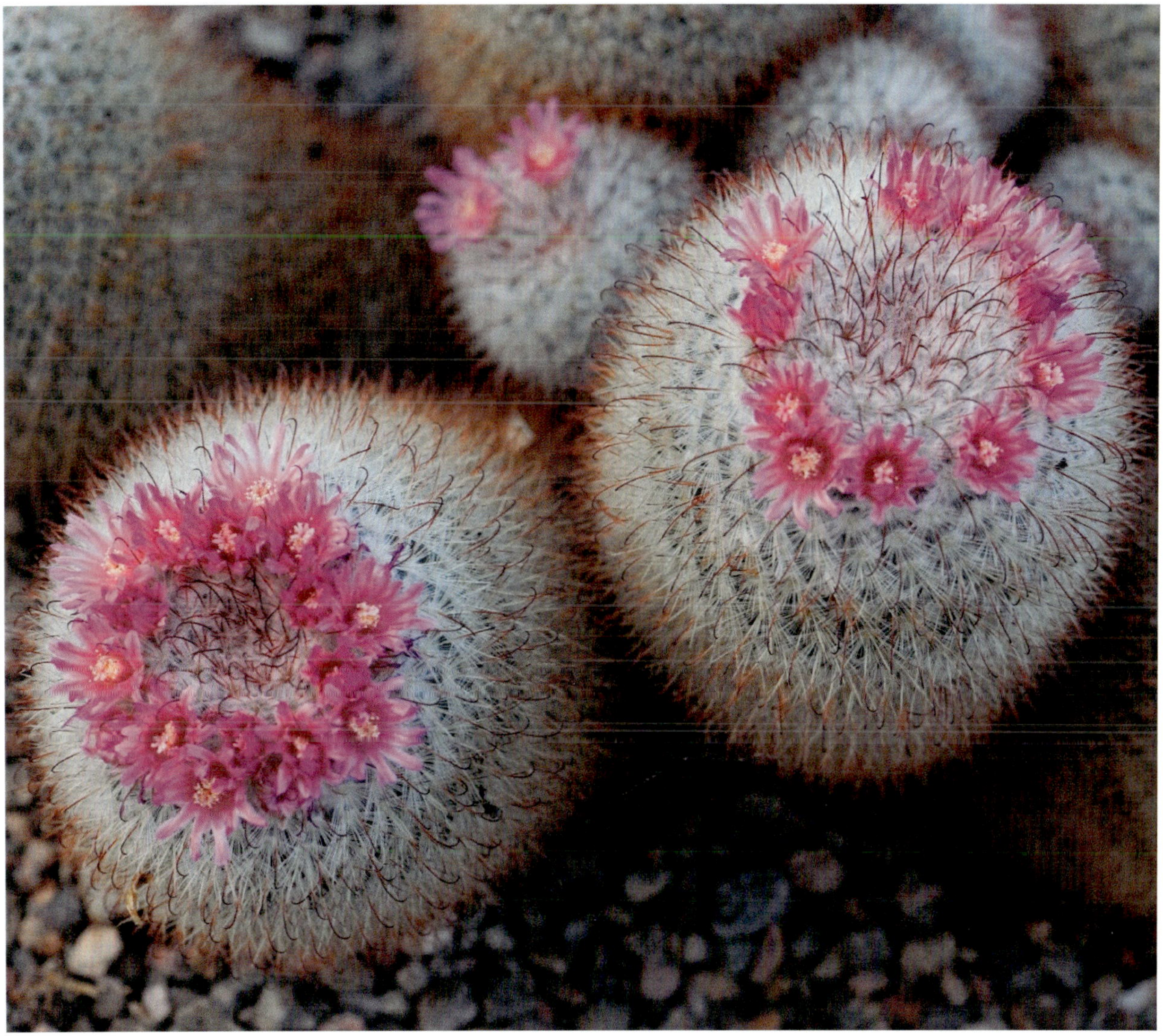

These pincushion cactus plants show off their tiny purple flowers.

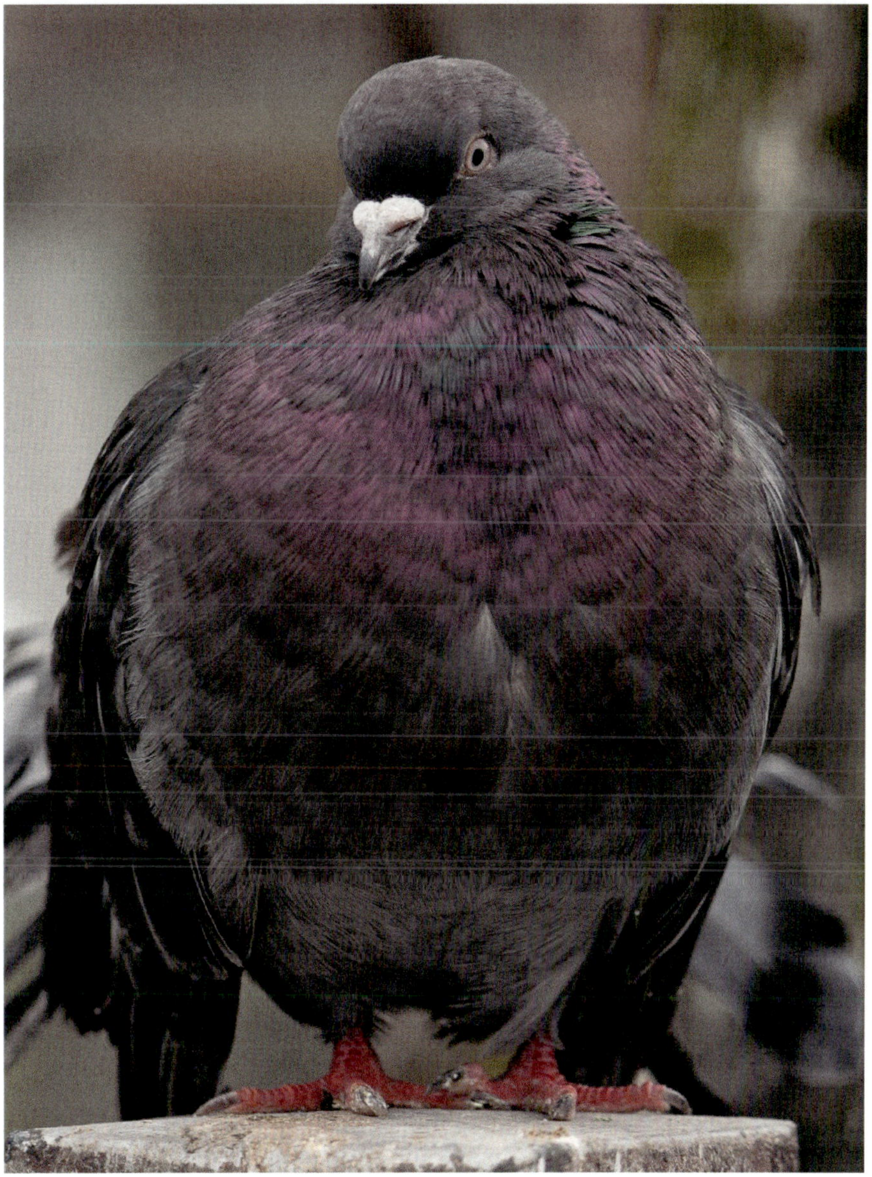

This beautiful bird is the Giant Homer pigeon.
The dark purple on his chest holds touches of green.

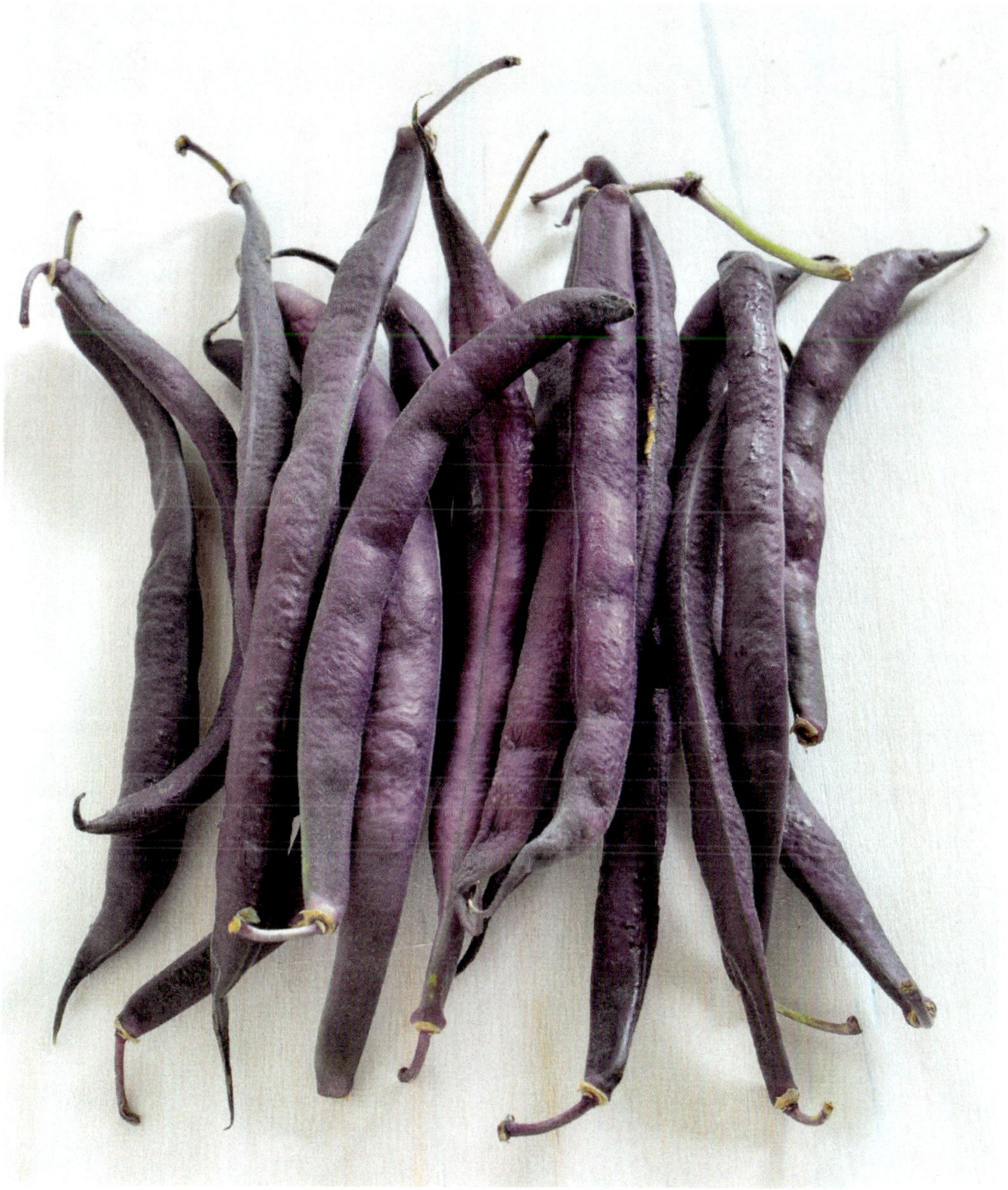

Purple wax beans turn green if cooked for over 2 minutes.

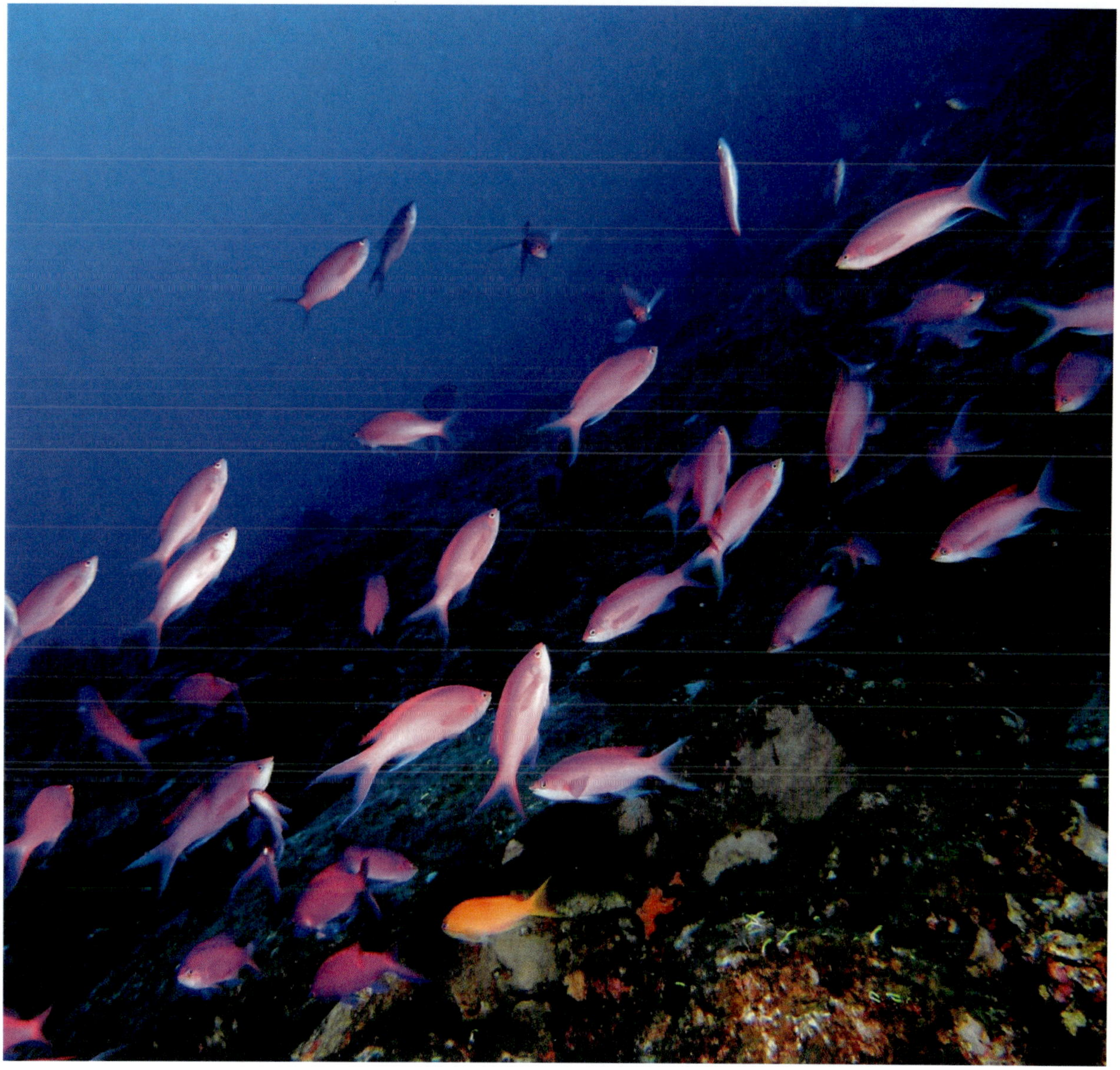

A school of Purple Queen fish swim in the Pacific Ocean.

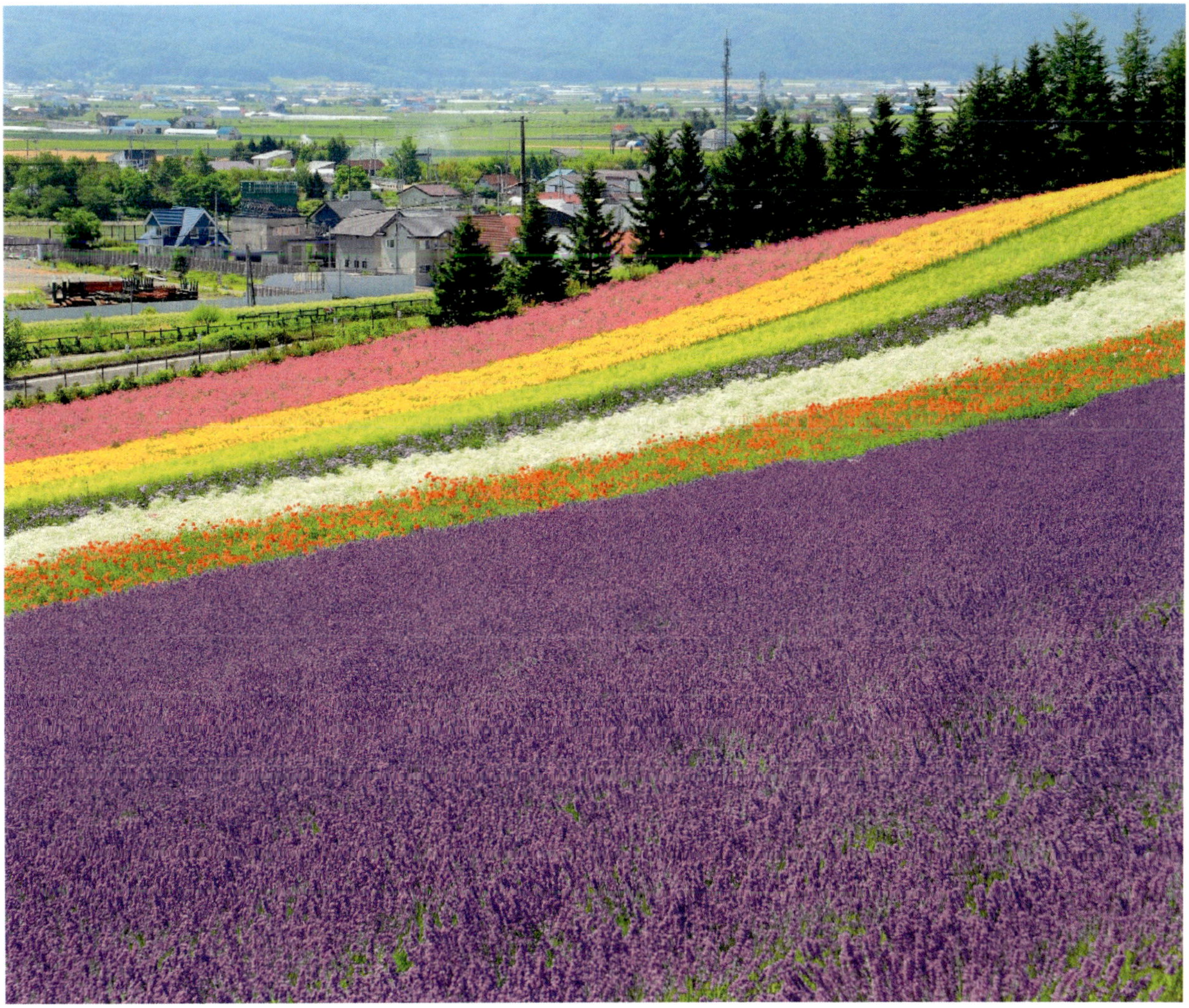

Purple lavender joins other fabulous colors
in this famous flower field in Japan.

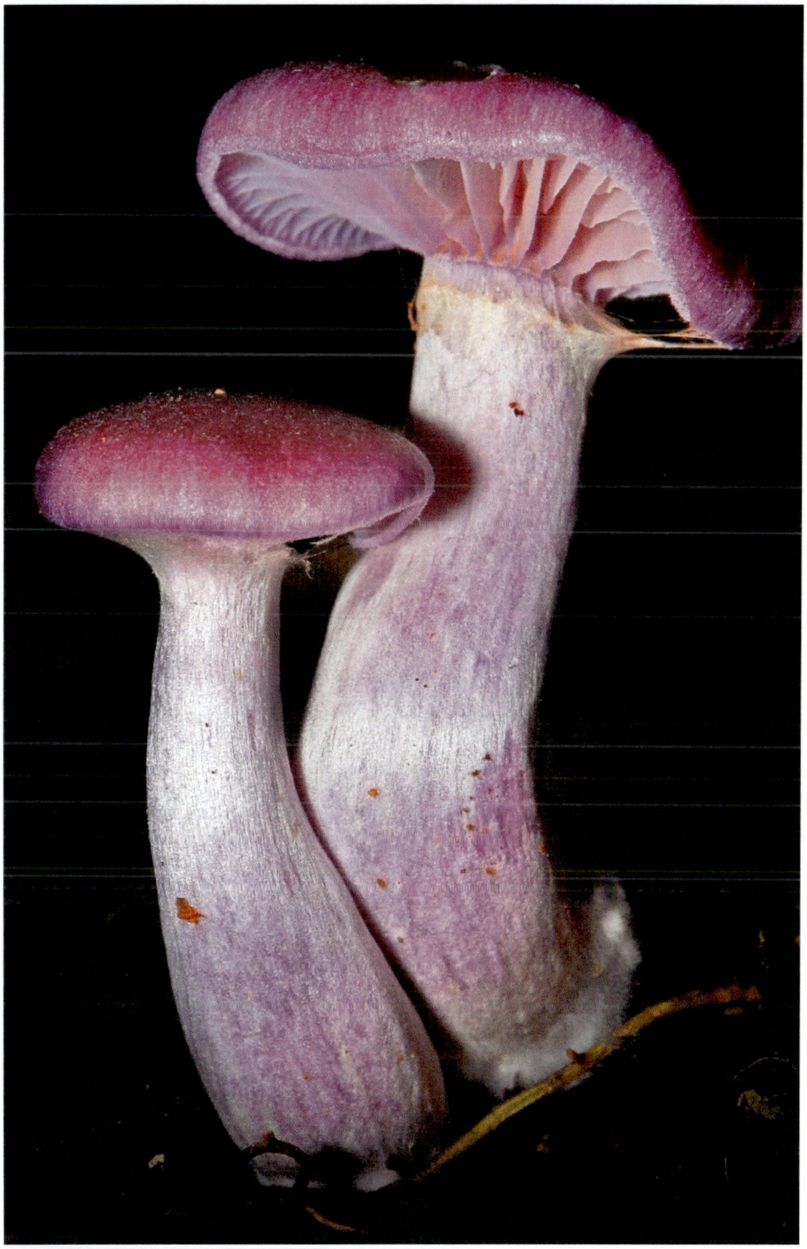

These pretty purple mushrooms grow on the floor of a rainforest in Malaysia.

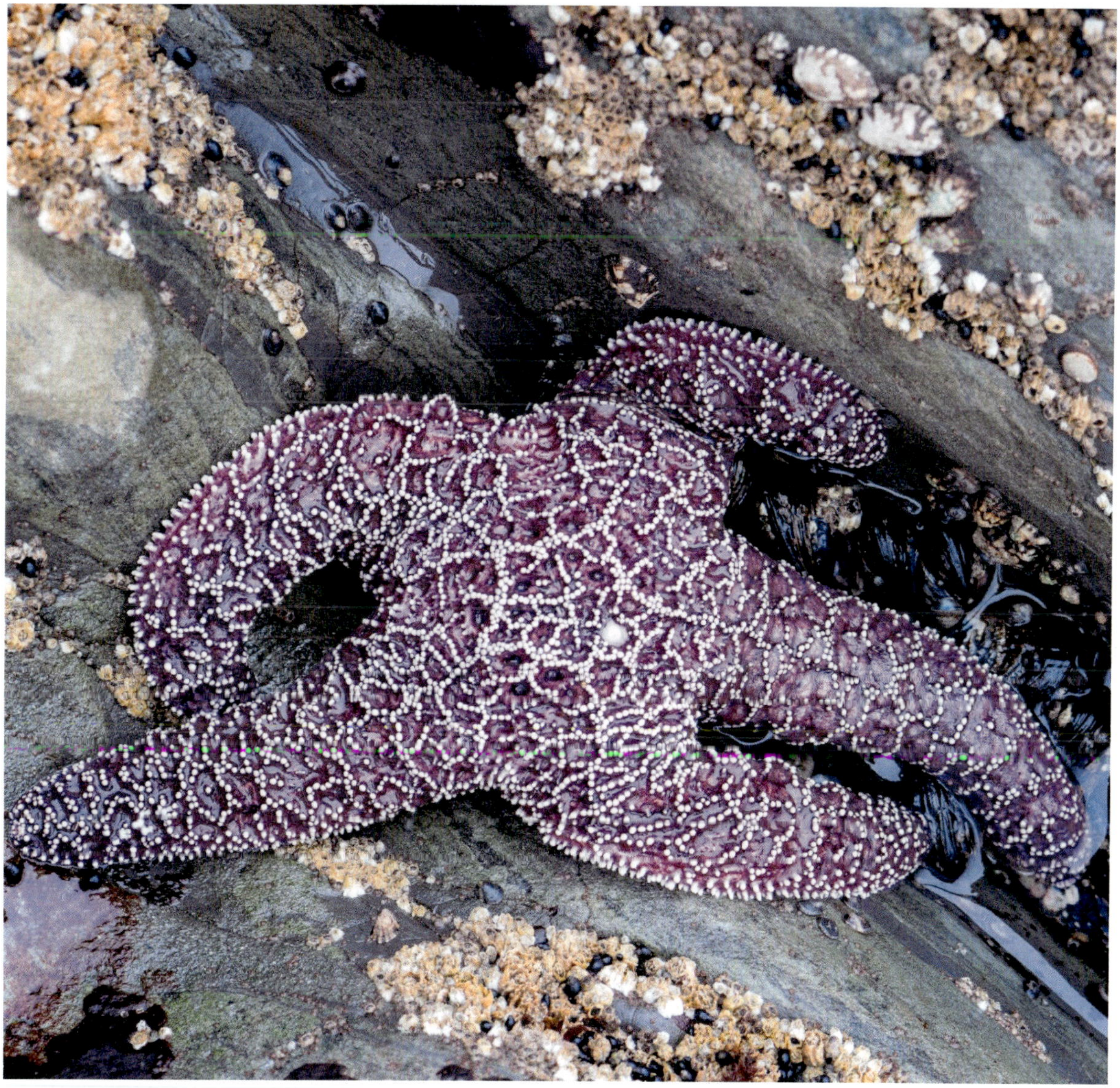

A beautiful dark purple starfish on the beach of Washington state.

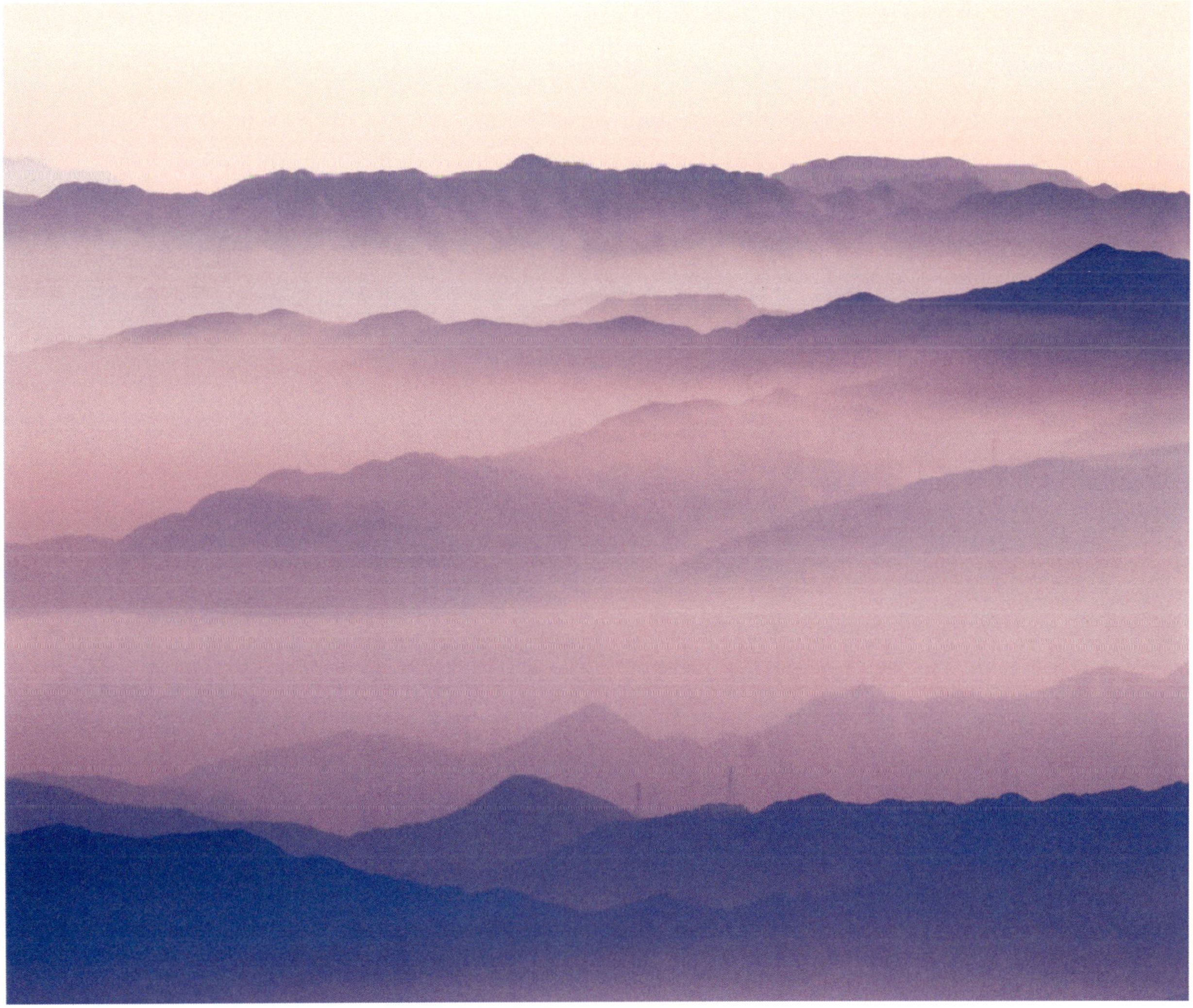

These Japanese mountain ridges display a spectacular purple haze.

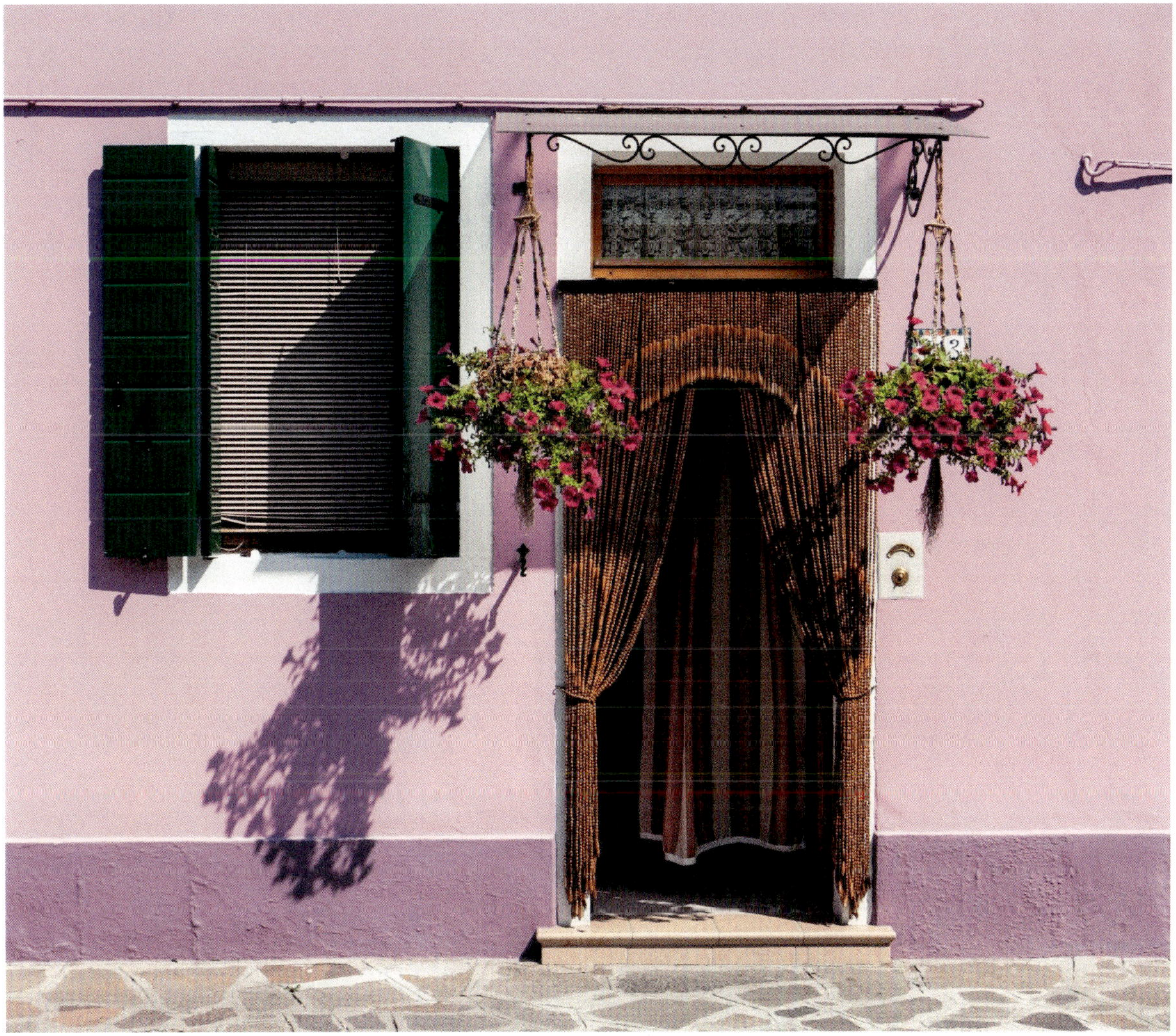

This colorful establishment, with its two-toned purple wall, is on the island of Burano, Italy.

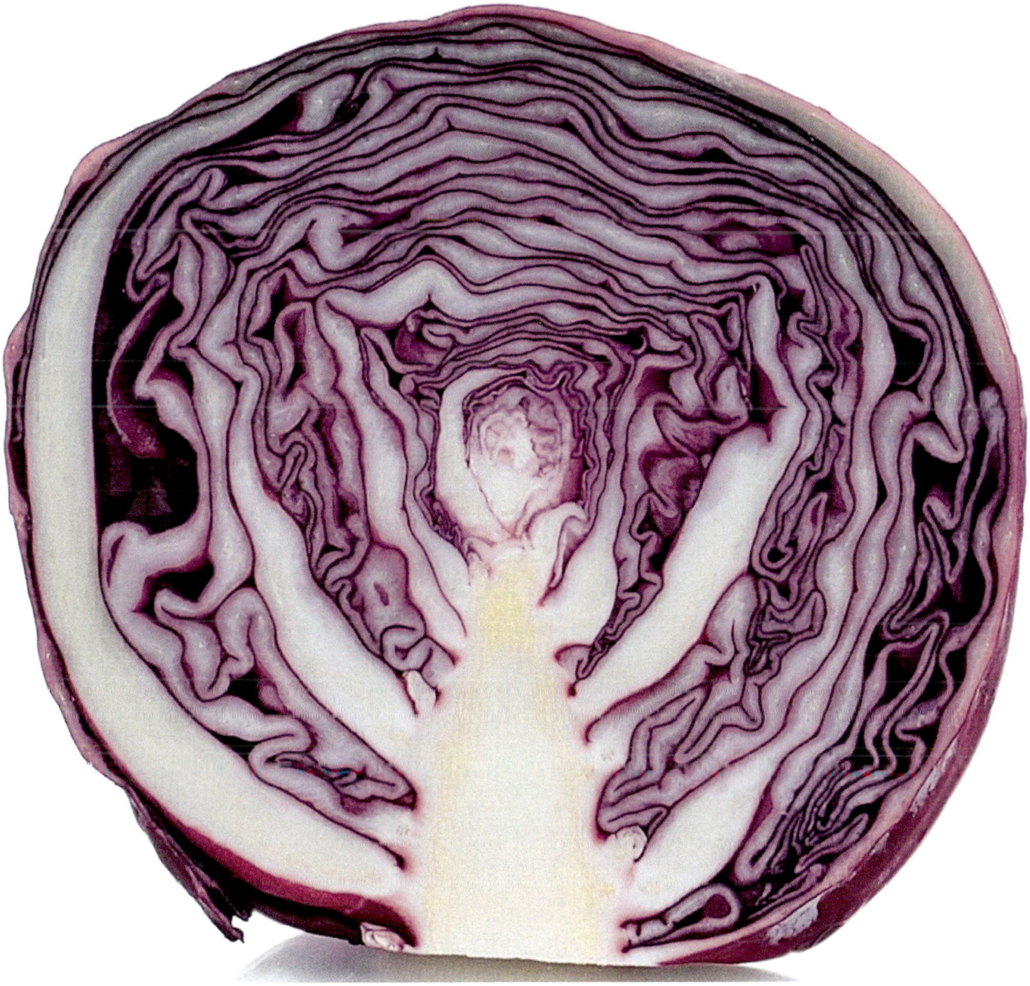

Close-up photo of the dark purple, intricate patterns of red cabbage.

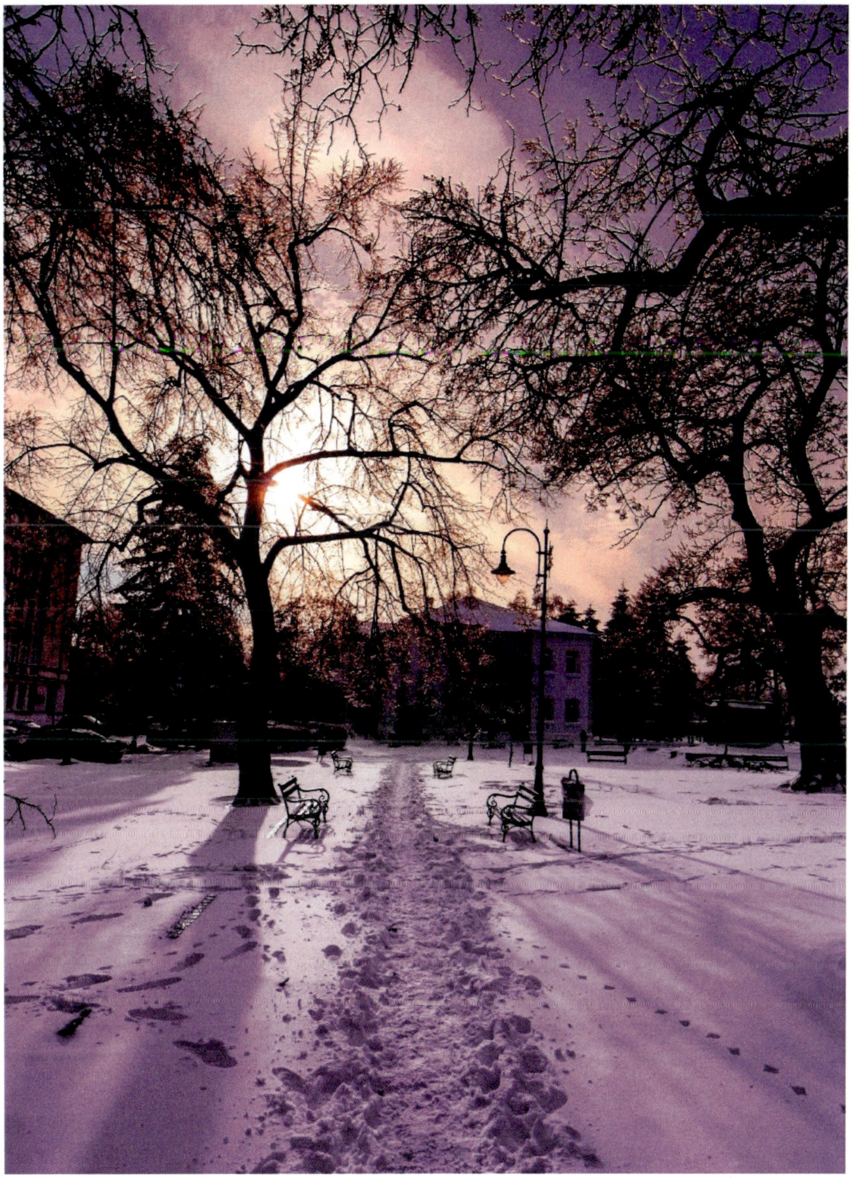

The setting sun casts a magical purple shimmer onto the snow in this Vermont town.

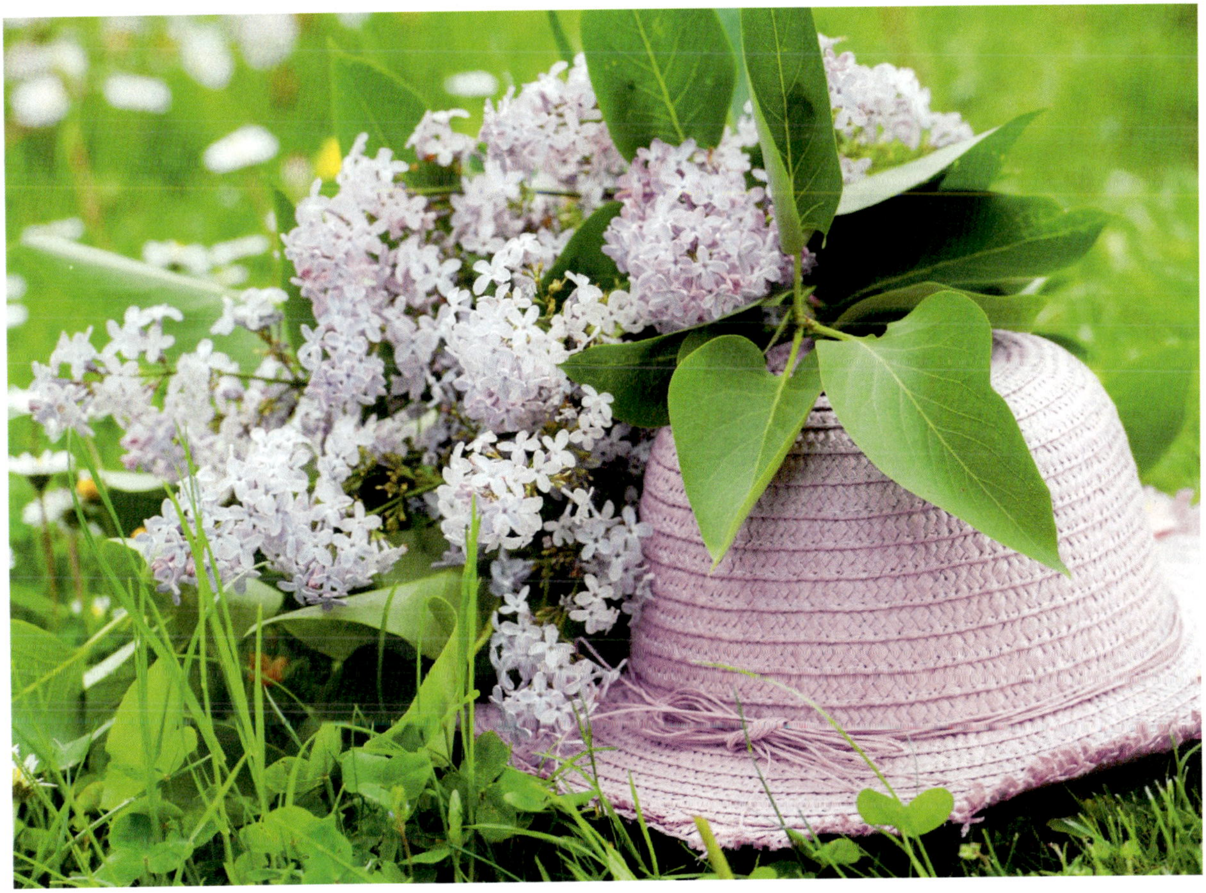

A pastel purple sunhat has found its perfect resting spot, next to this bouquet of lilacs.

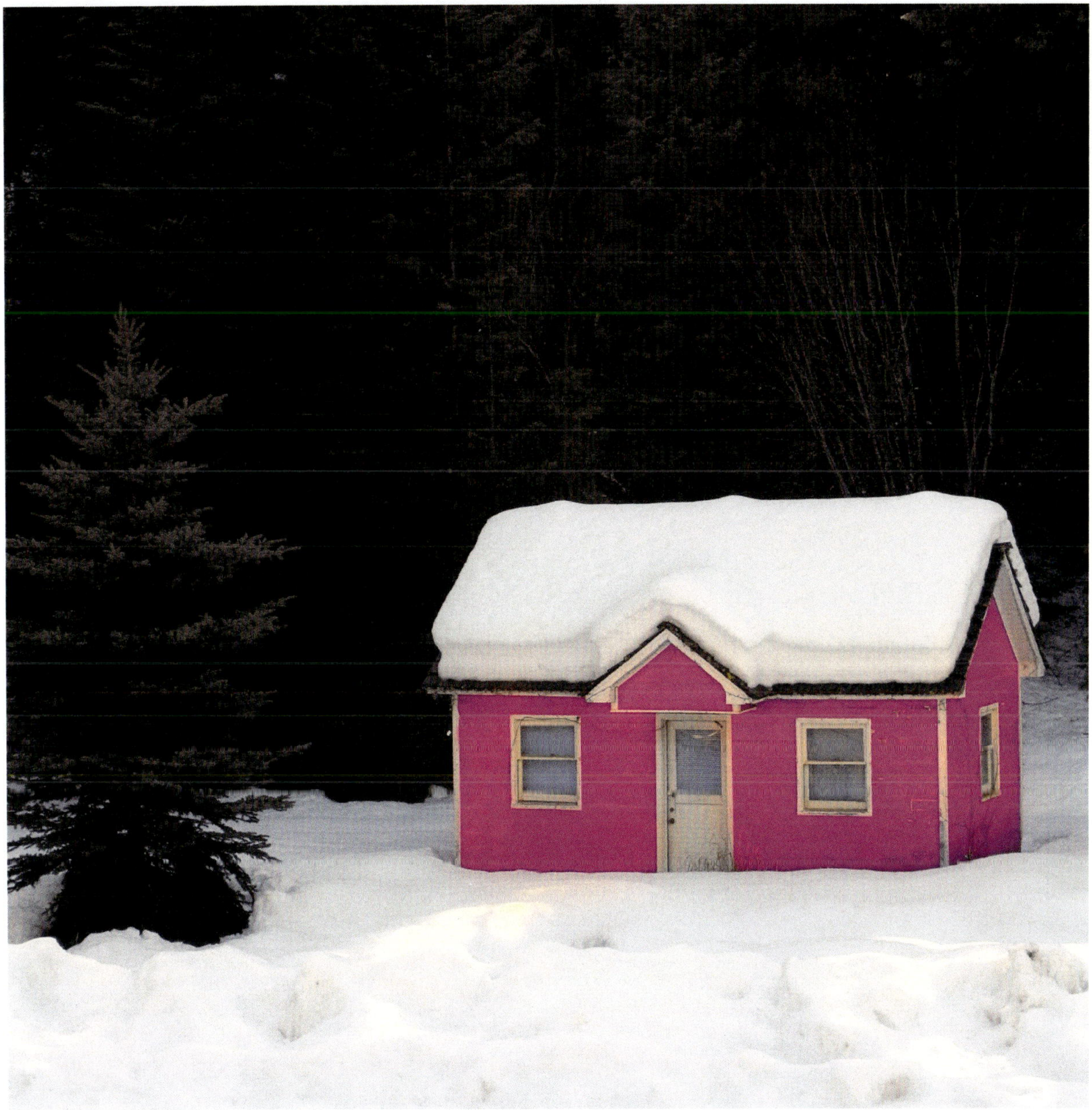

Heavy snow blankets this bright purple tiny home.

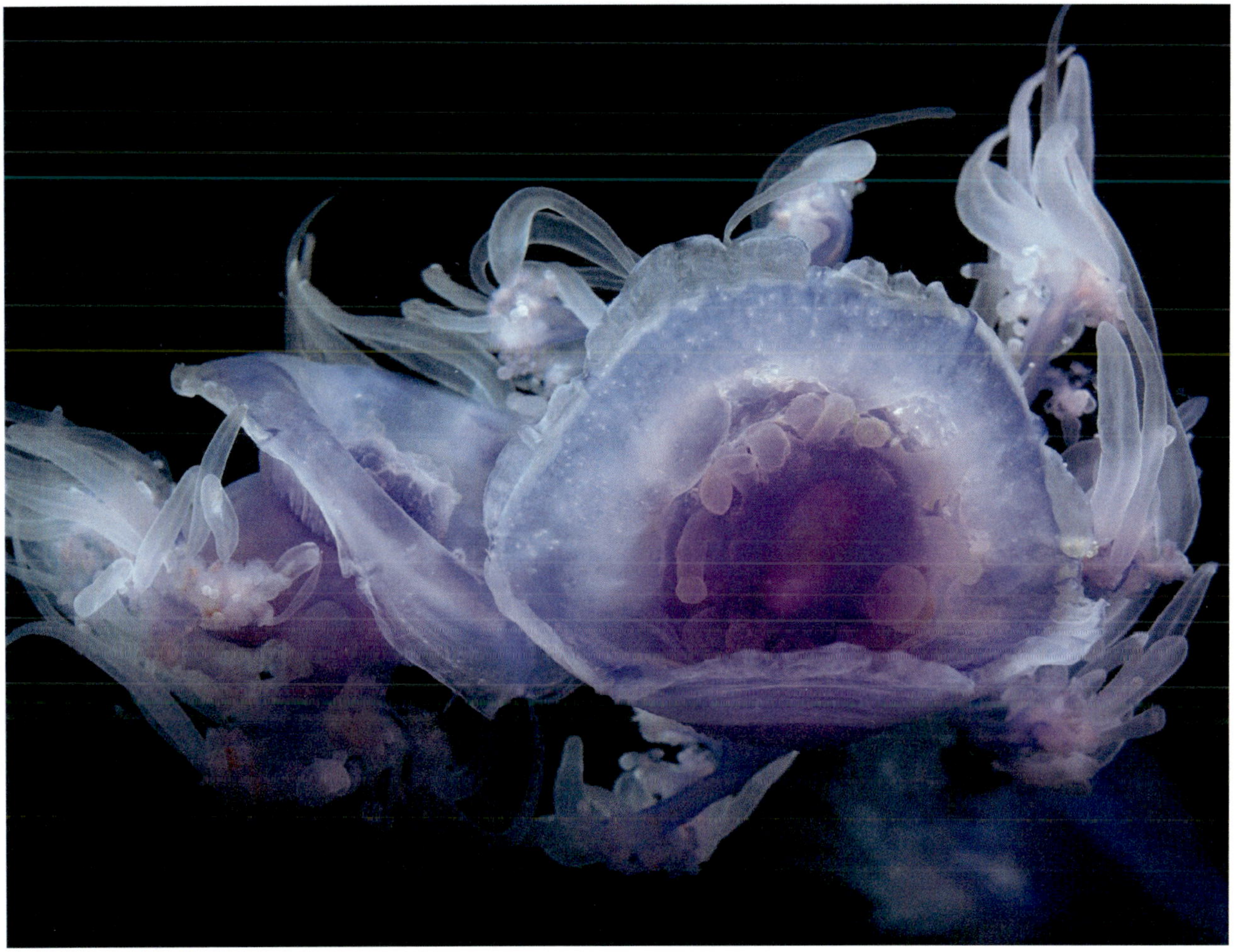

The colorful Crown Jellyfish has shimmering blues and purples.

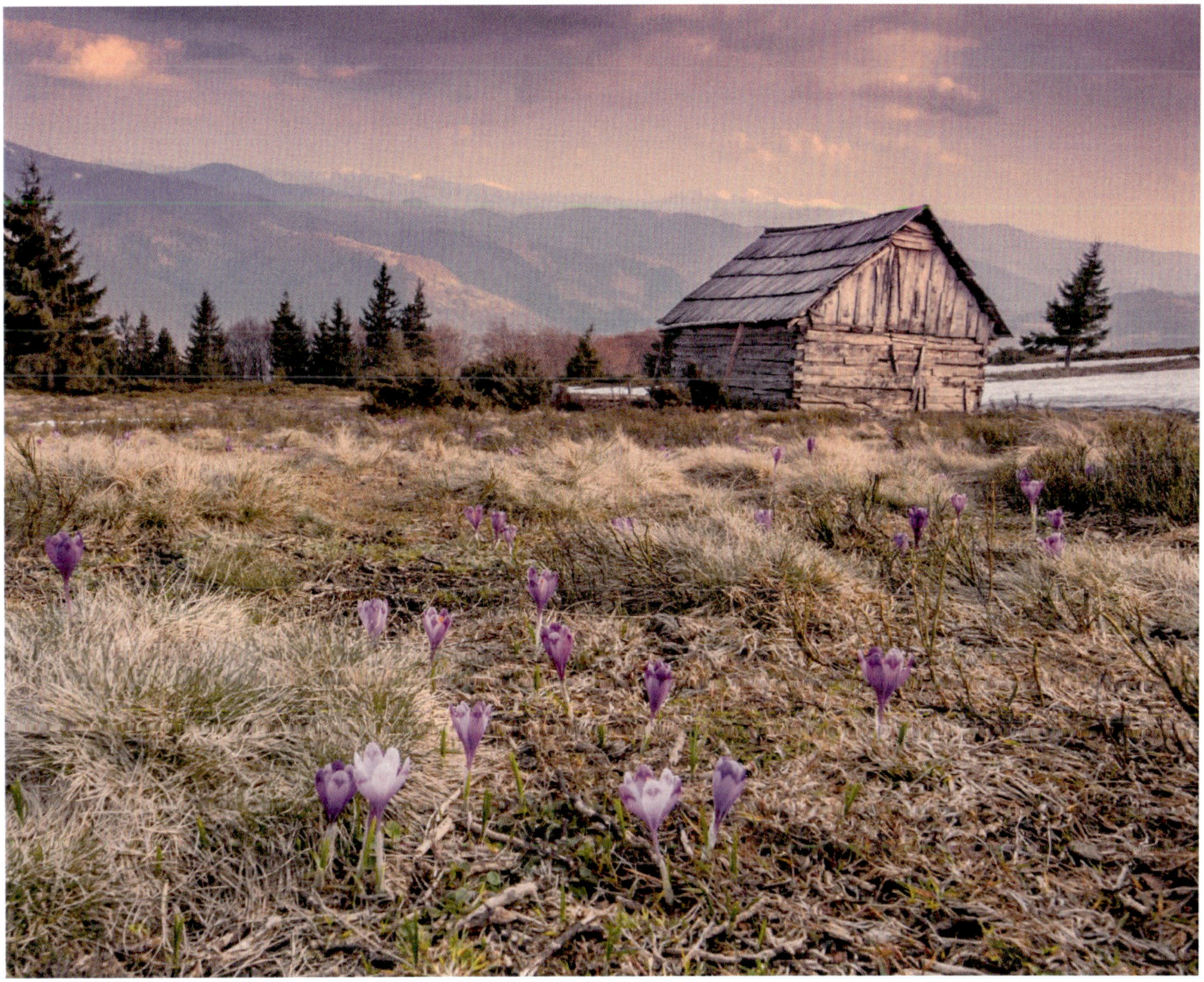

Purple crocus flowers add a perfect pop of color to the scenery of this old wooden house in front of sweeping mountains.

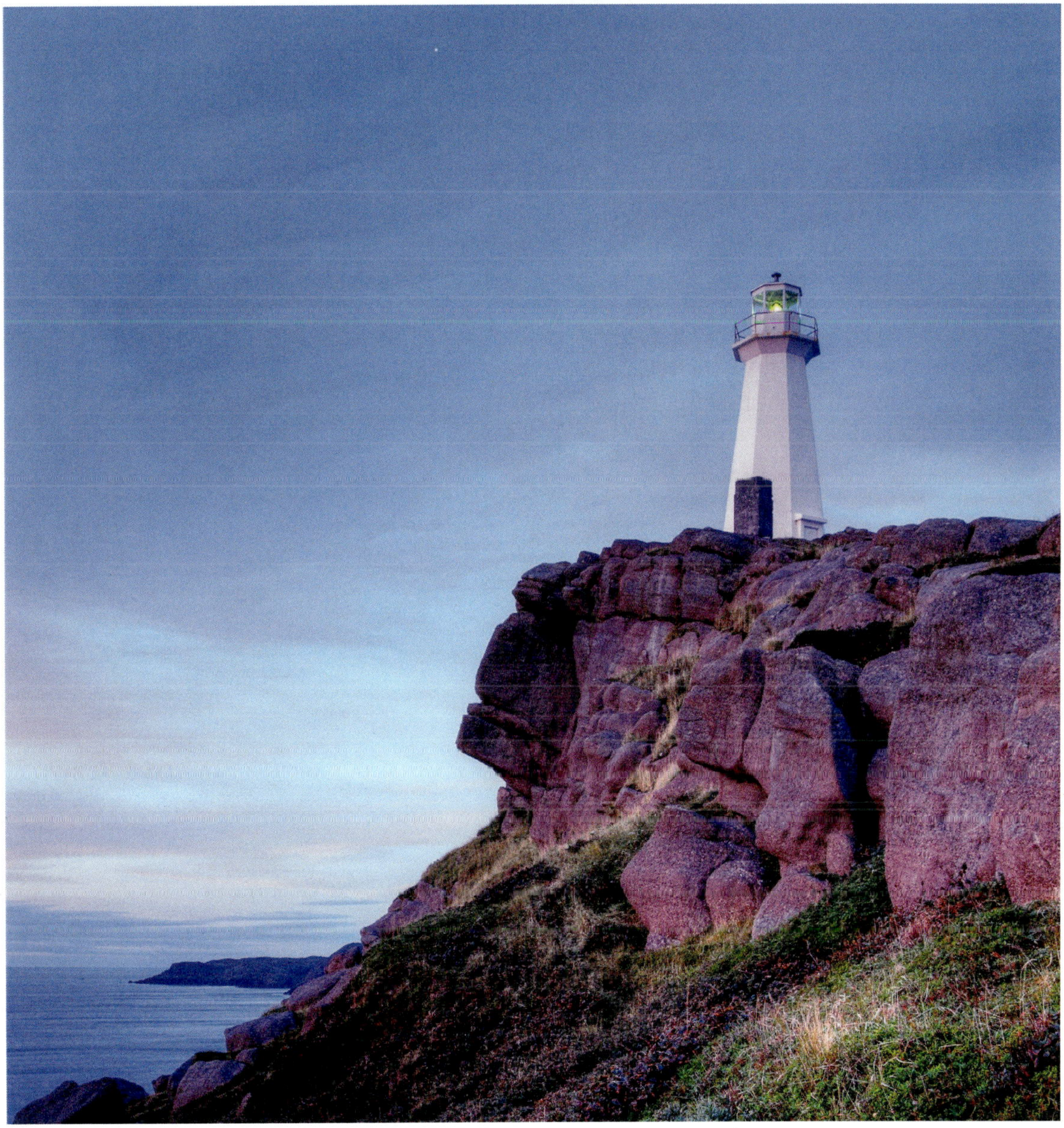

The Cape Spear lighthouse stands proud atop dark purple cliffs in Newfoundland, Canada.

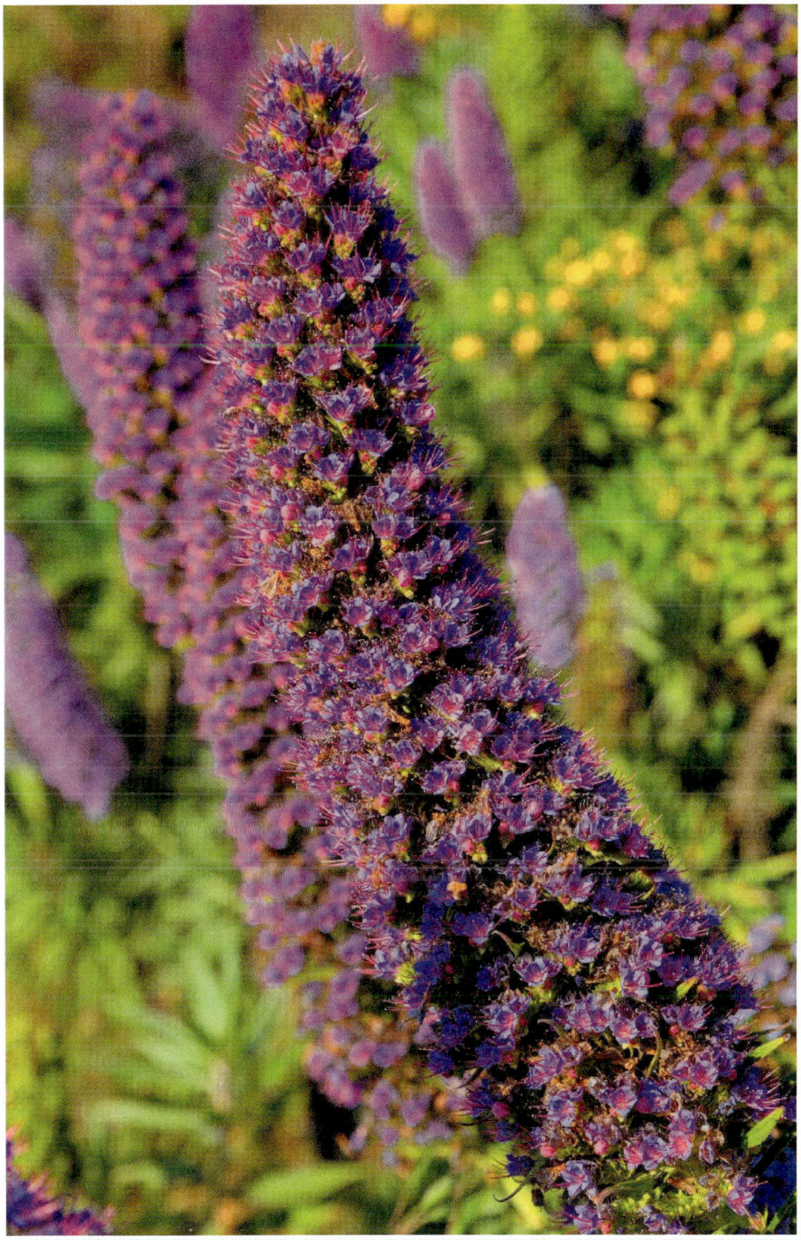

These purple flowers are called Pride of Madeira.

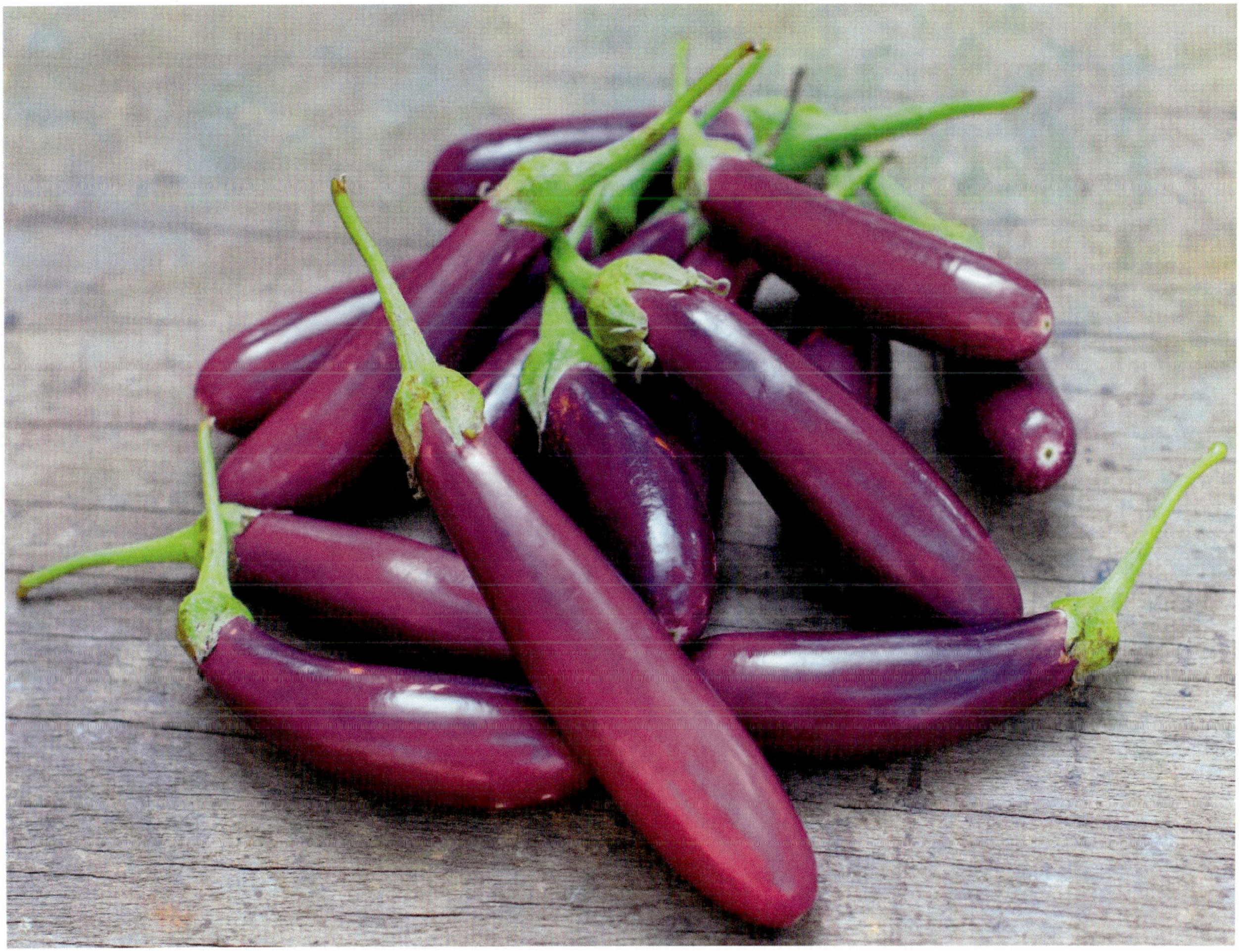

A pile of freshly picked purple eggplants.

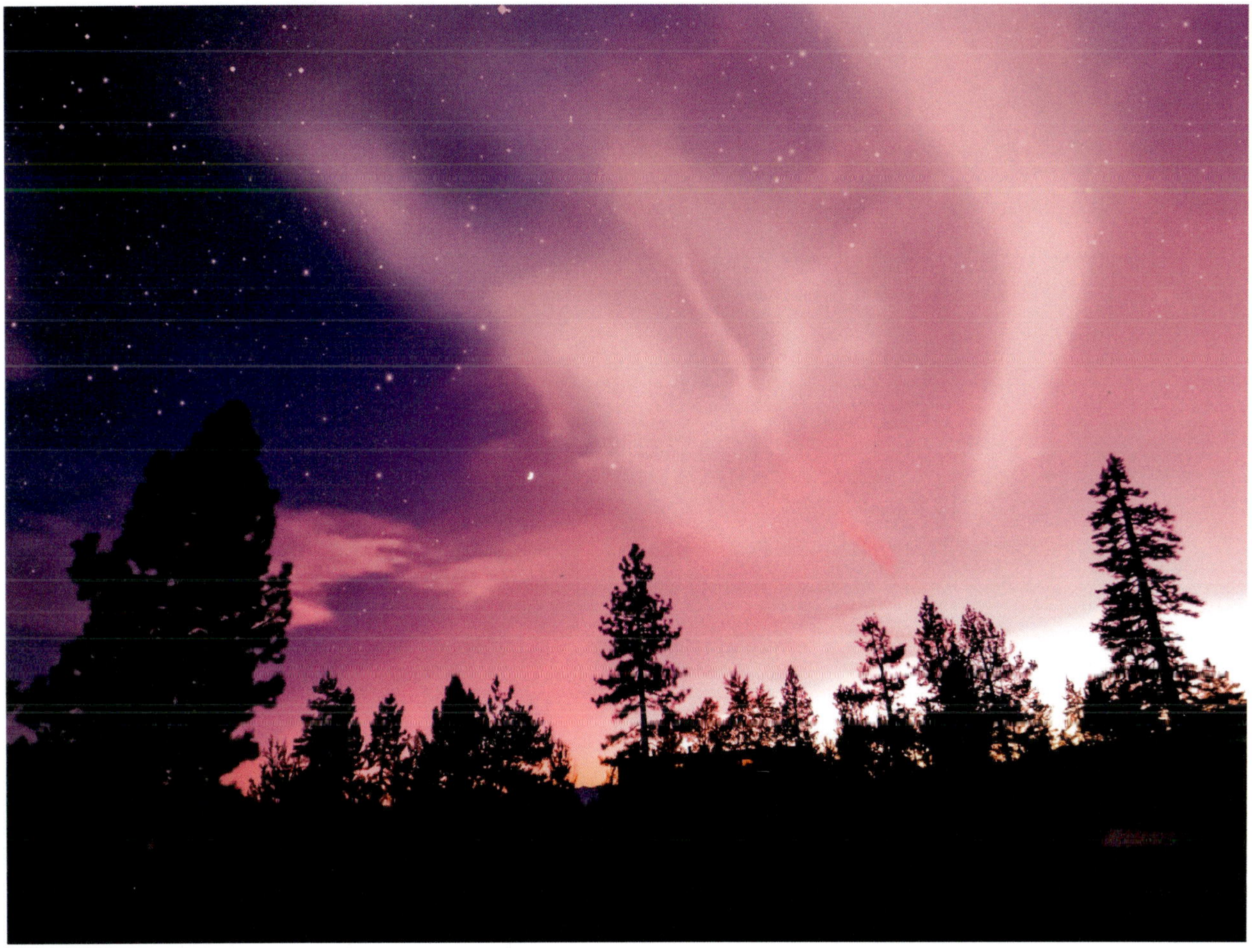

A spectacular purple and pink display of the Northern Lights in Alaska.

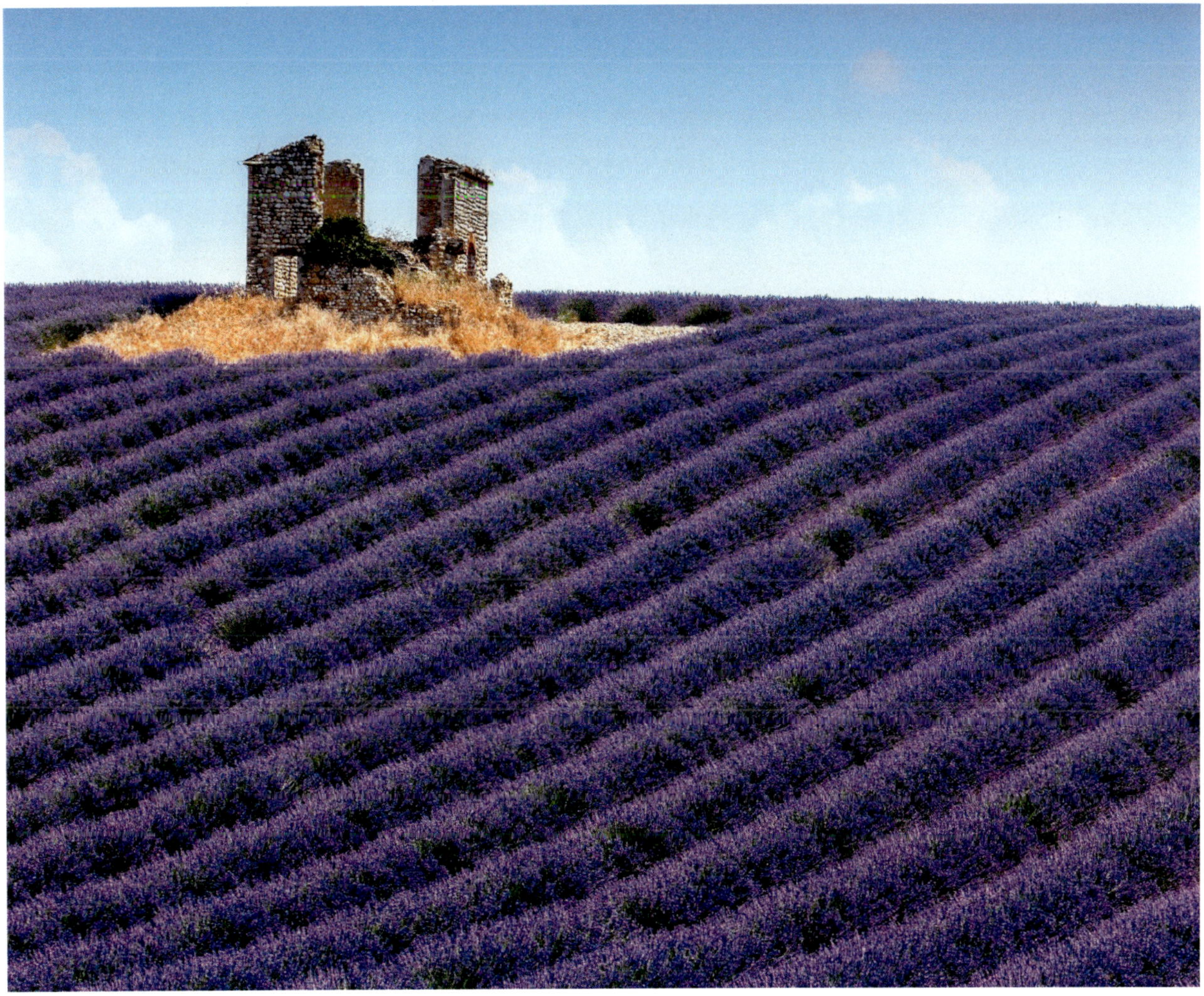

Lush lavender fields create a purple carpet around the ruins of a castle in France.

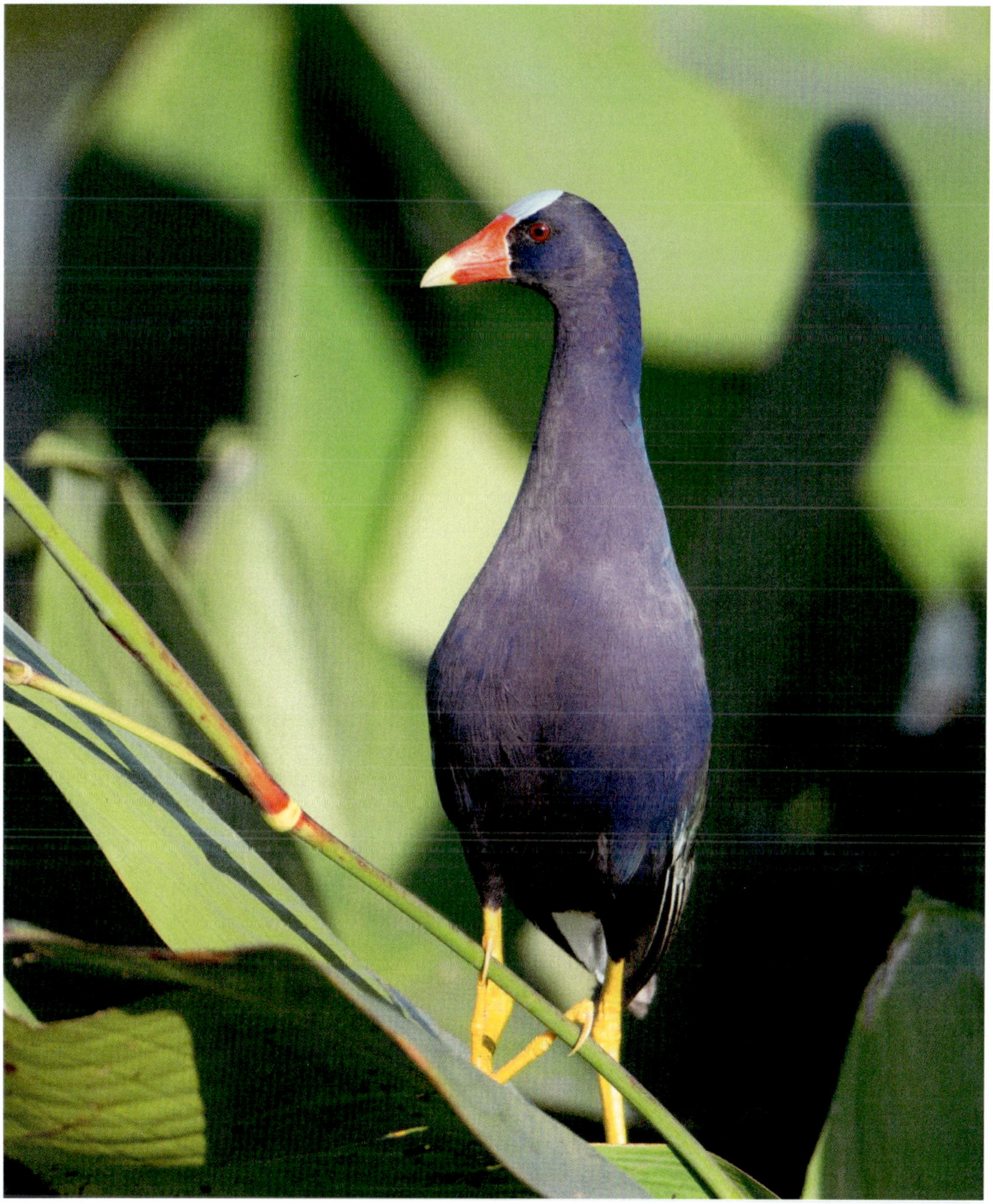

The Purple Gallinule bird is common in south Florida.

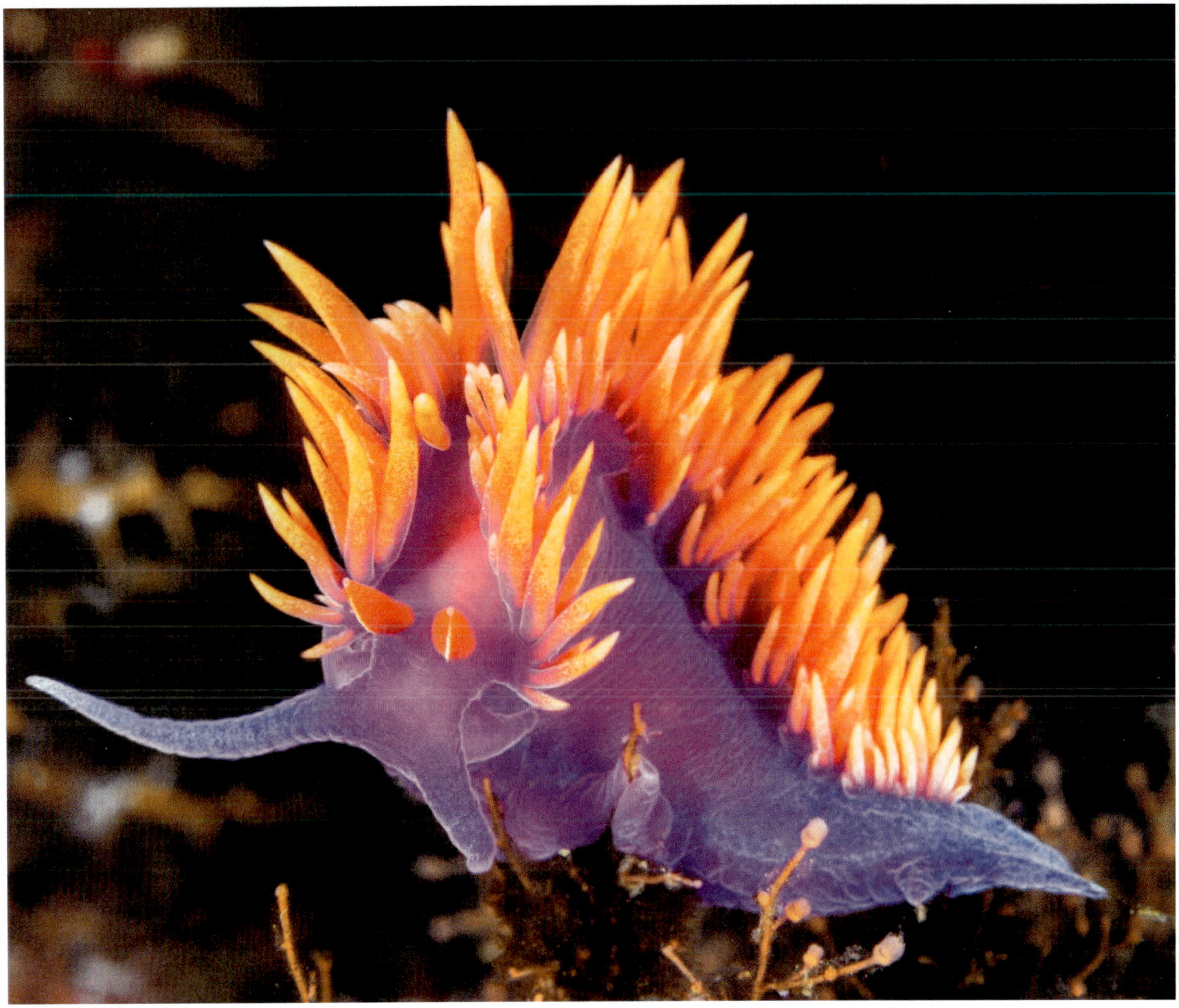

This amazing purple and orange creature is a snail.
It is called the Spanish Shawl.

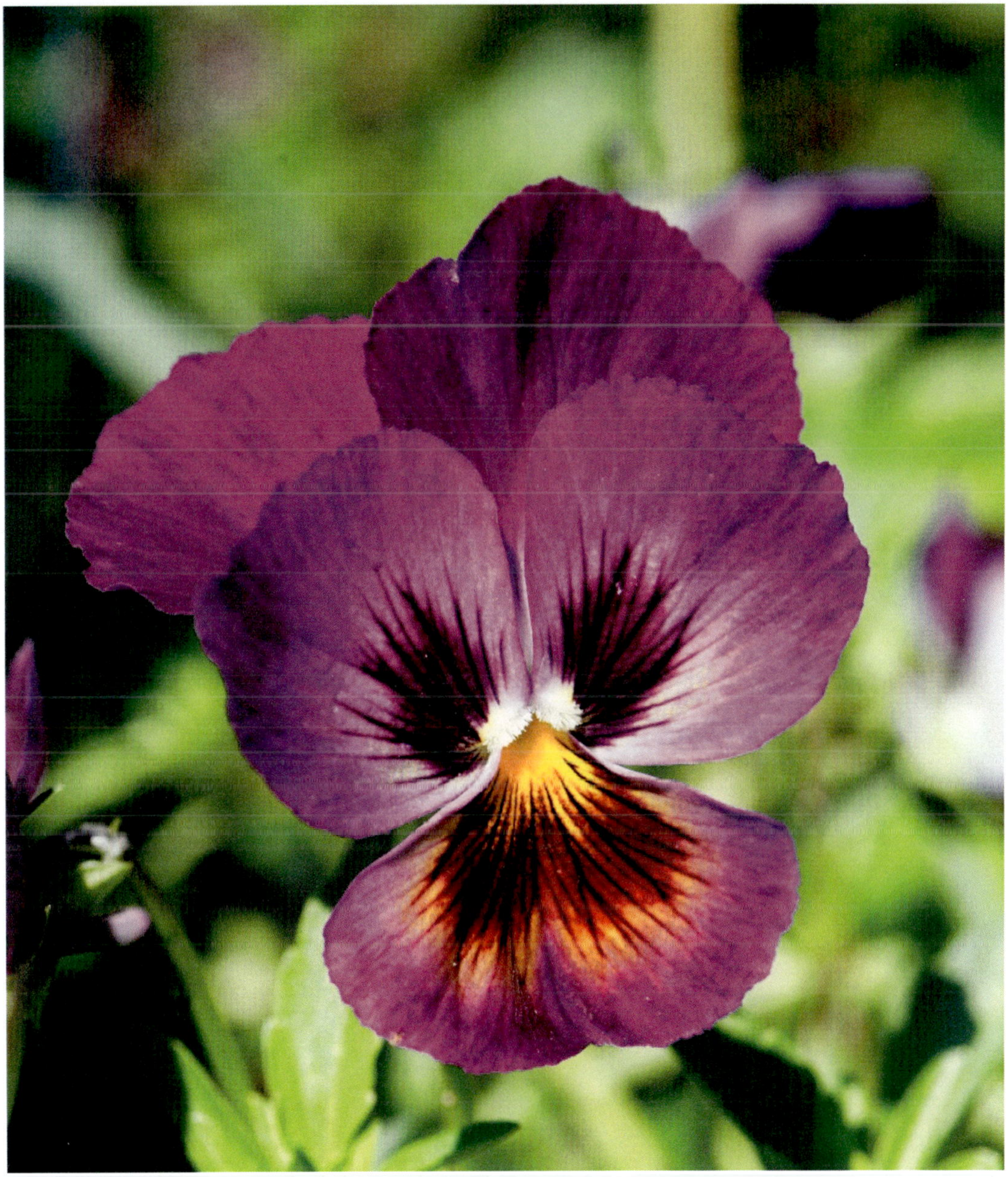

Close up photo of the eye-catching purple pansy flower.

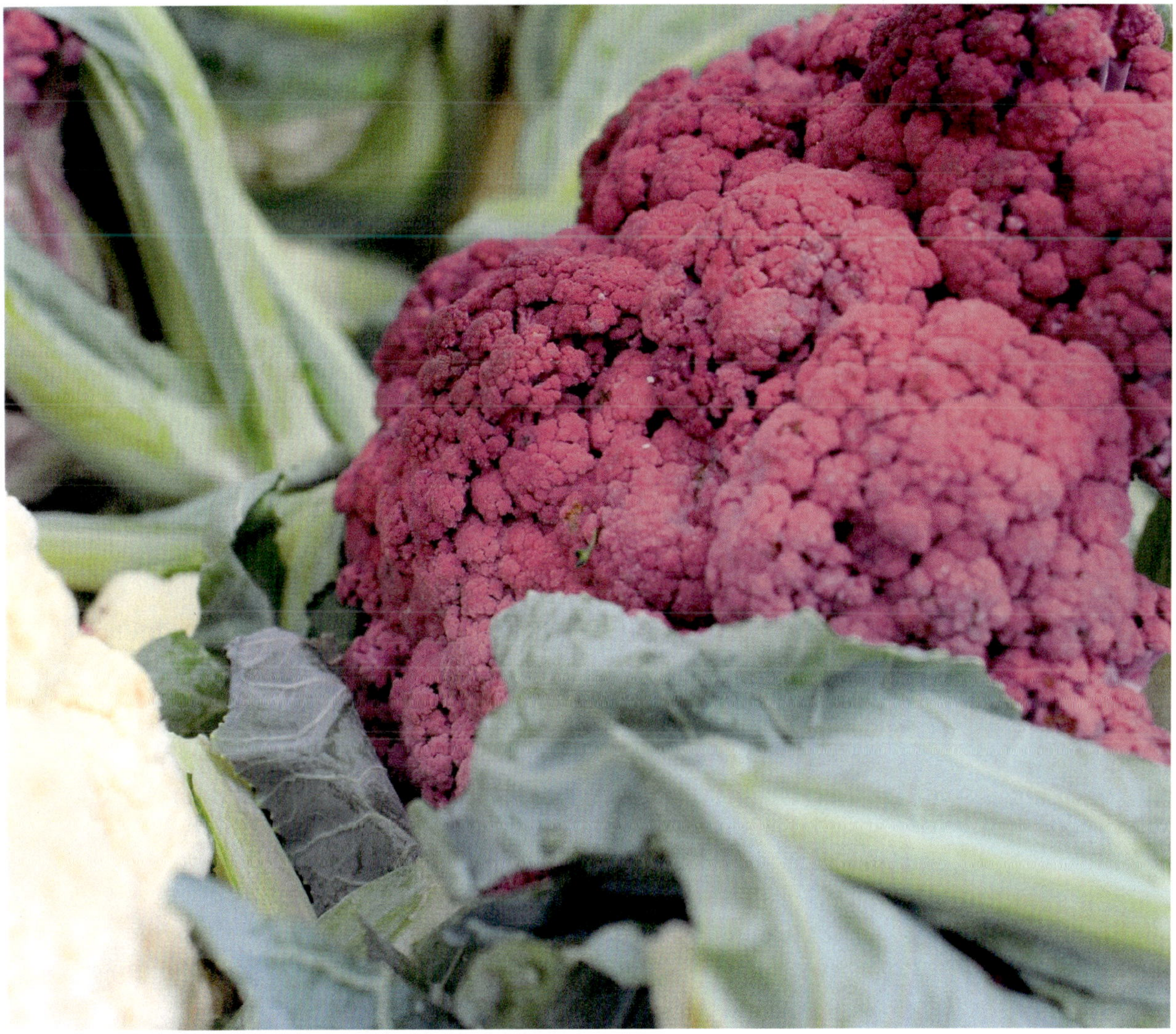

Purple cauliflower is a sought-after treat at local farmer's markets.

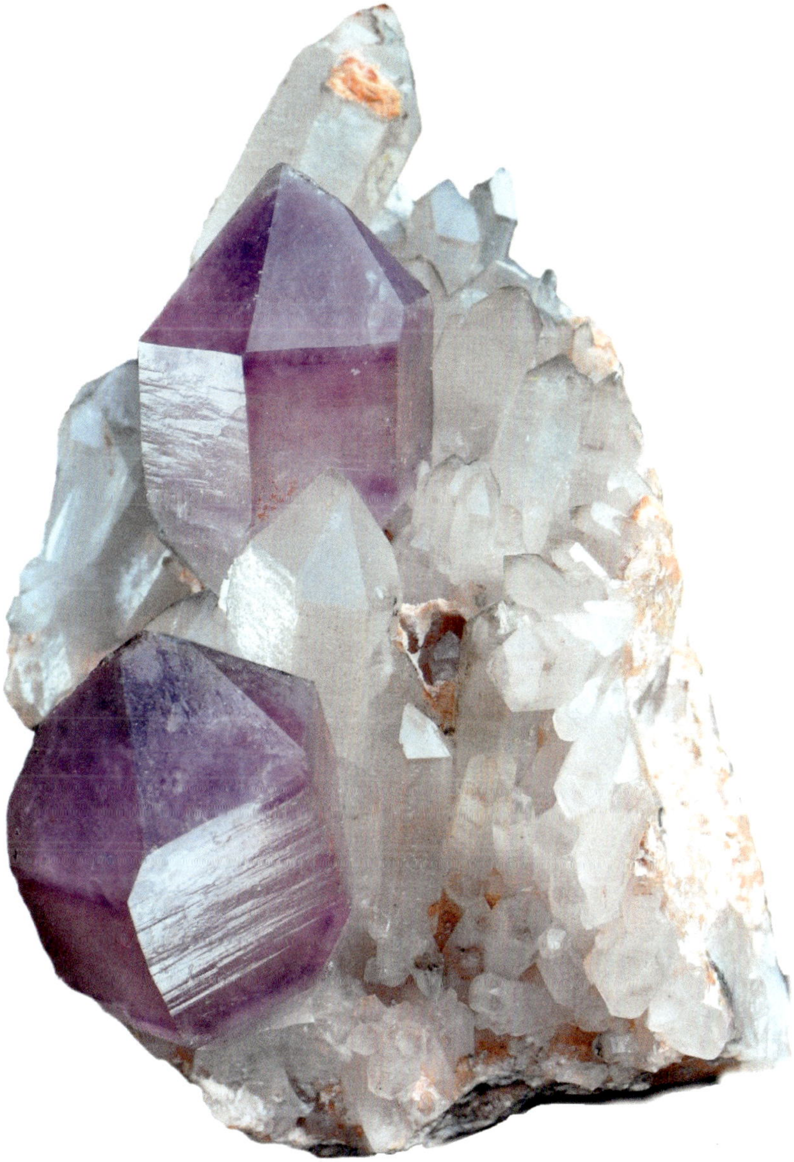

The purple you see here is Amethyst, a violet variety of quartz.

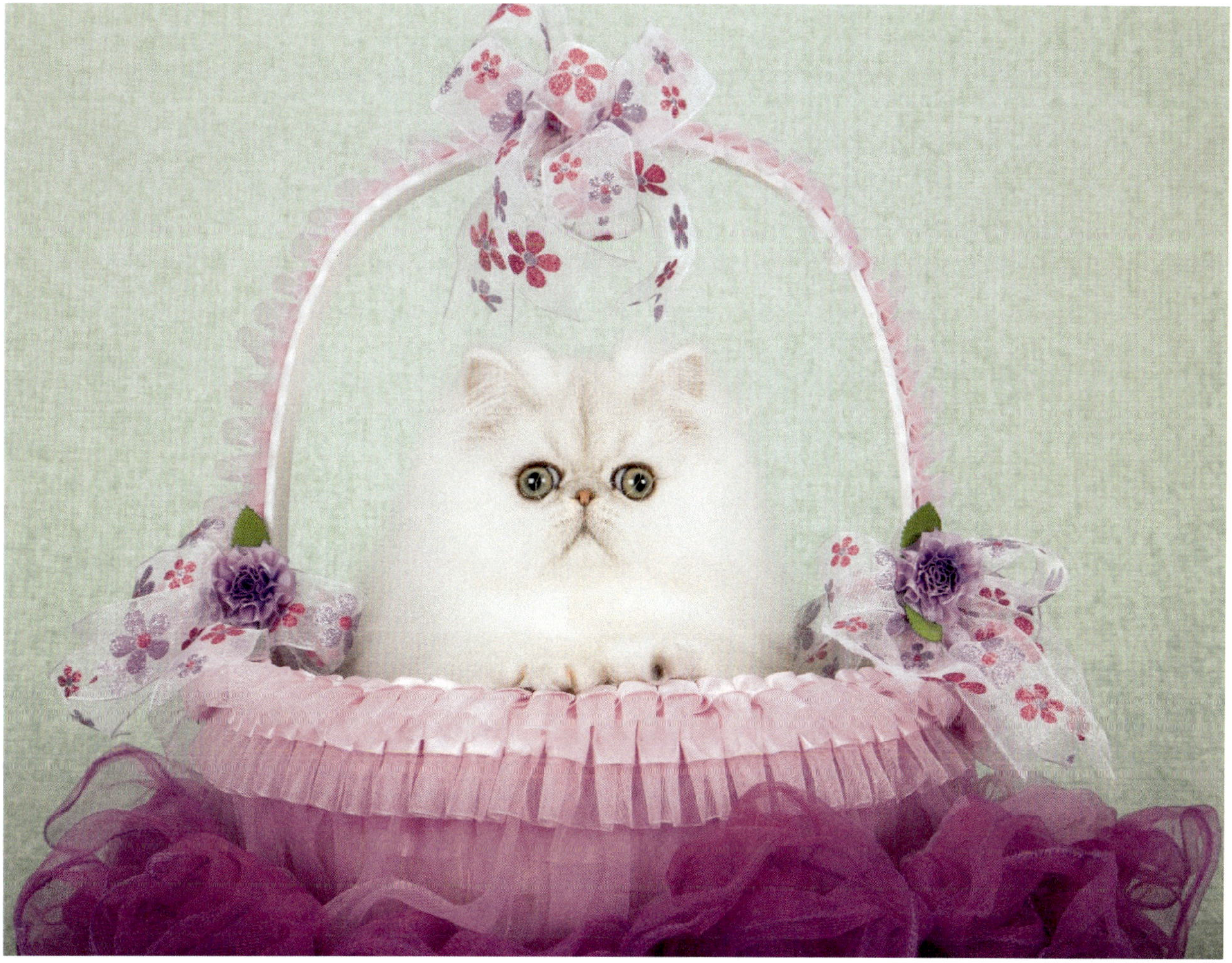

A Silver Chinchilla kitten sits inside an artfully decorated purple basket.

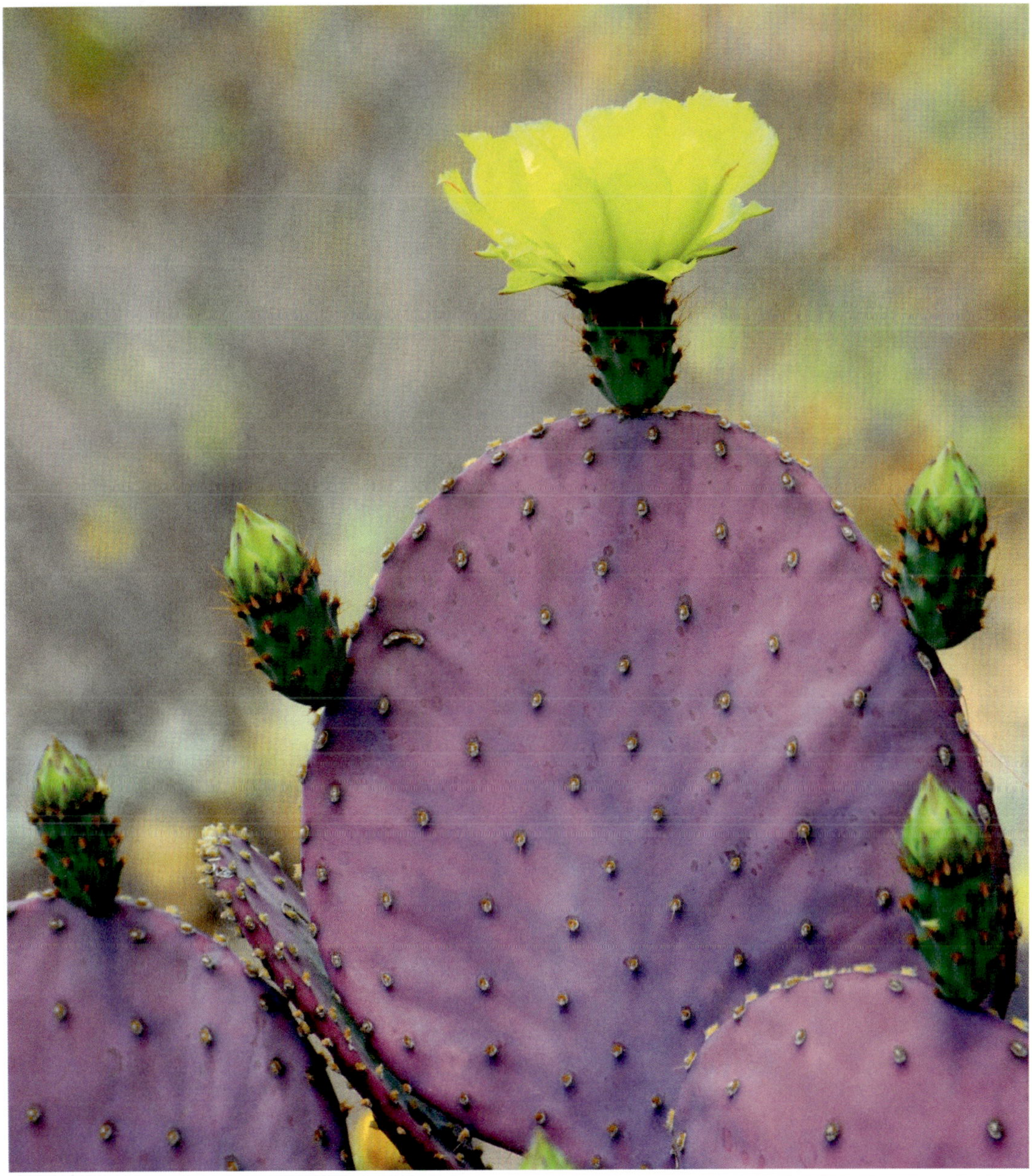

A purple leaf prickly pear cactus in bloom.

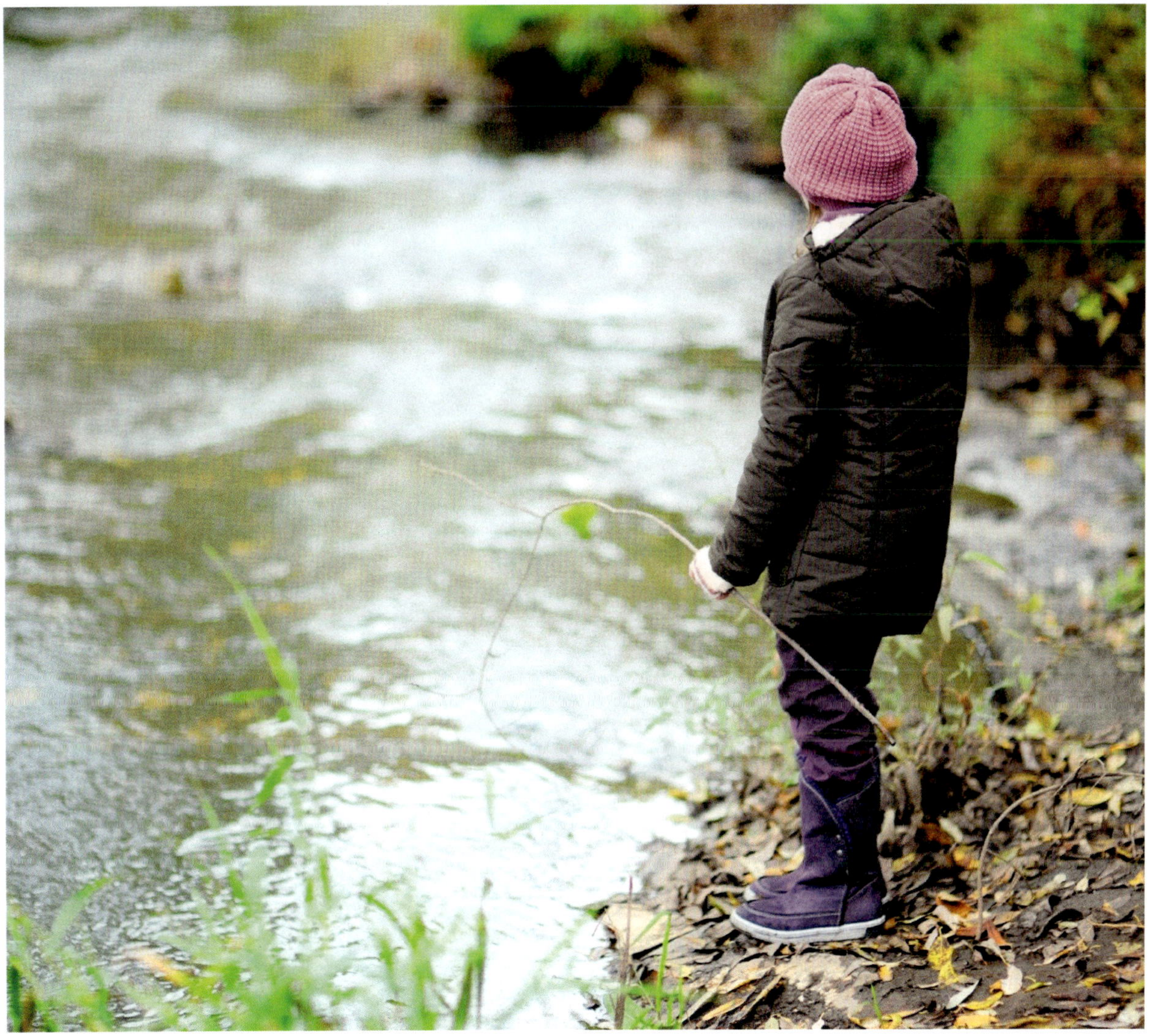

A young girl with a purple hat watches the dancing waters of a river in New Hampshire.

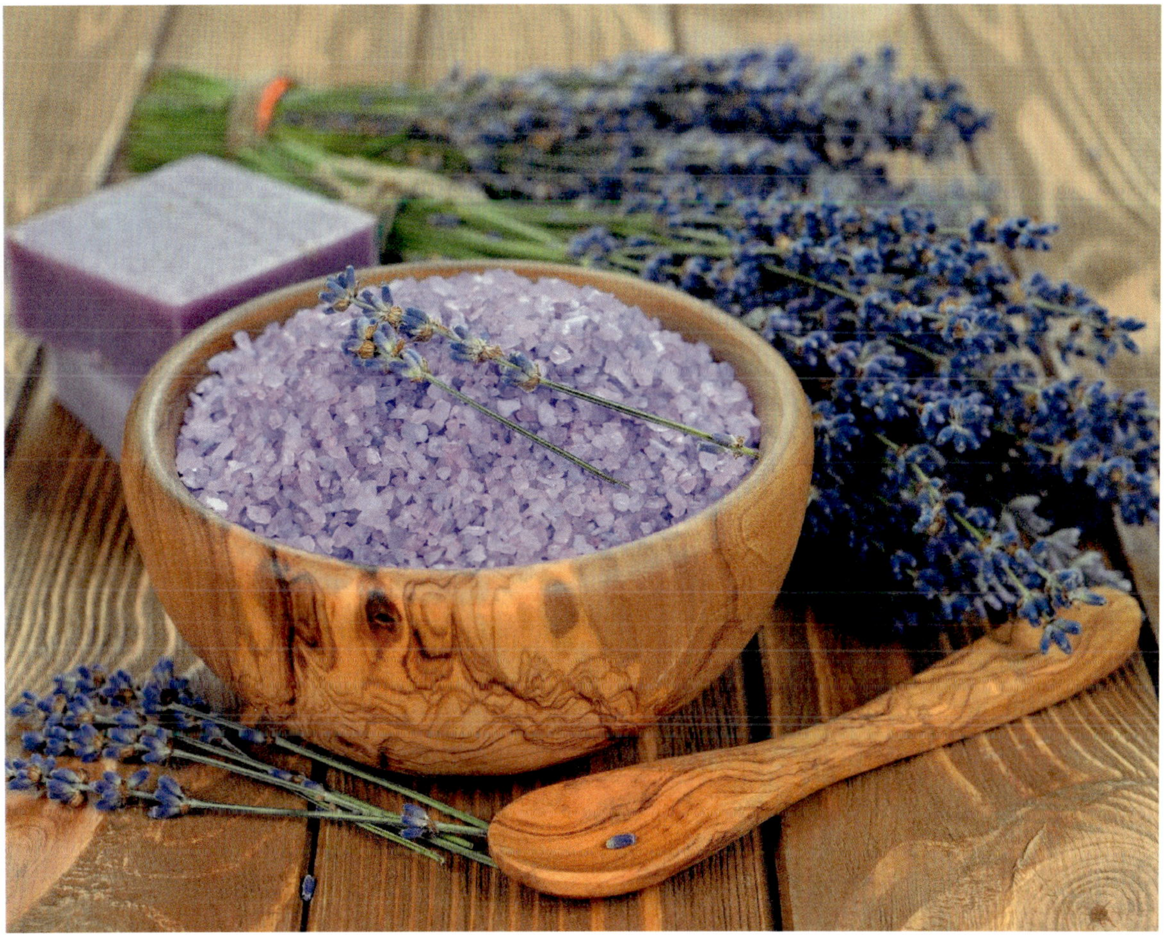

Purple sea salt has been prepared on a table decorated with cut lavender.

OTHER BOOKS IN THIS SERIES BY EMMA ROSE SPARROW

A Bevy of Blue

A Year's Worth of Yellow

A Gathering of Green

A Parcel of Purple

A Reservoir of Red

A World of White

An Ocean of Orange

Photo Credits

The artist/source credits for the photos in this book are listed in the order in which they appear:

Lucia Pitter/Shutterstock.com
Benjamin Sime/Shutterstock.comneta
Willie Davis/Shutterstock.com
Eva Gruendemann/Shutterstock.com
Linda Hughes/Shutterstock.com
Vilainecrevette/Shutterstock.com
JeniFoto/Shutterstock.com
Gaby Kooijman/Shutterstock.com
Henrik Larsson/Shutterstock.com
Cosmin Manci/Shutterstock.com
Axel Jauer/Shutterstock.com
aastock/Shutterstock.com
Ellen Mol/Shutterstock.com
Oleg Znamenskiy/Shutterstock.com
cohlmann/Shutterstock.com
Jung Hsuan/Shutterstock.com
David HAJES Hajek/Shutterstock.com
brackish_nz/Shutterstock.com
photogal/Shutterstock.com
Masahiro Suzuki/Shutterstock.com
littlewormy/Shutterstock.com
Ryan M. Bolton/Shutterstock.com
Nagel Photography/Shutterstock.com
YuryZap/Shutterstock.com
LYSVIK PHOTOS/Shutterstock.com
amphaiwan/Shutterstock.com
KingJC/Shutterstock.com
Dora Zett/Shutterstock.com
Lane V. Erickson/Shutterstock.com
Ken Wolter/Shutterstock.com
Smit/Shutterstock.com
ggw1962/Shutterstock.com
holbox/Shutterstock.com
CHAIWATPHOTOS/Shutterstock.com
SurangaSL/Shutterstock.com
andre@cf/Shutterstock.com
Dennis W. Donohue/Shutterstock.com
Joe Belanger/Shutterstock.com
Kucher Serhii/Shutterstock.com
OryGonian/Shutterstock.com
Albert Russ/Shutterstock.com
Linn Currie/Shutterstock.com
AHPix/Shutterstock.com
Alinute Silzeviciute/Shutterstock.com
Olyina/Shutterstock.com

17882217R00058

Made in the USA
Middletown, DE
28 November 2018